Adrift

Adrift

*fieldnotes from
almost-motherhood*

MIRANDA WARD

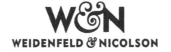

WEIDENFELD & NICOLSON

First published in Great Britain in 2021 by Weidenfeld & Nicolson
an imprint of The Orion Publishing Group Ltd
Carmelite House, 50 Victoria Embankment
London EC4Y 0DZ

An Hachette UK Company

1 3 5 7 9 10 8 6 4 2

A CIP catalogue record for this book is
available from the British Library.

ISBN (Hardback) 978 1 4746 1415 3
ISBN (eBook) 978 1 4746 1417 7

Typeset by Input Data Services Ltd, Somerset
Printed in Great Britain by Clays Ltd, Elcograf S.p.A.

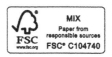

www.weidenfeldandnicolson.co.uk
www.orionbooks.co.uk

For my grandmother

Contents

One

On the Cusp

2013–2014

I

A Matter of Time

I am in the library, looking something up, and there it is.

A swimming pool. A blue rectangle, divided into sixths by five vertical white lines; a flash of sunbleached green at the top of the shot, a concrete path running out of view, the thin brown trunks of a scattering of trees just visible, extending the verticality of the white lines.

I lean close to read the caption. *Pool #6*, part of Ed Ruscha's series *Nine Swimming Pools and a Broken Glass* (1968). The lines are what hold my attention: they are straight, they are true; they lead the gaze from the bottom to the top of the photograph, and then off, out, beyond. They seem, too, to contain something, though the pool itself is empty, or perhaps it's that they seem to form the basis for something. (The line as *conduit, a boundary, an exacting / course of thought*, as the poet Matt Donovan puts it: *Surface engraved with a narrow stroke, path / imagined between two points*.) They are – to me – what gives everything else structure. They offer a starting point, a path along which to travel, a way of making sense.

Ruscha, born in Nebraska, moved to California in 1956 and has lived there ever since. His work, particularly his photography from the 1960s and 1970s, demonstrates an enduring interest in the vernacular landscapes of southern California and the American West more broadly: gas stations, parking lots, swimming pools. *Nine Swimming Pools and a Broken Glass* appeared first as a limited-edition photobook in 1968, though the images were printed in a separate portfolio in 1997. The book contains only ten photographs – of the nine pools and, finally, a broken glass tumbler on a blue background. But it is sixty-four pages long, most of the images separated by a seemingly irregular rhythm of blank pages. As if anything could happen in the spaces in between. As if to echo the blankness of the pools themselves, or the blank space signified by them, the possibility – and the constraint – their form suggests.

As if to say *something*, or perhaps *nothing*. As if—

*

When Alexander and I decided to have a baby I was young. We were not yet married. I had recently begun a PhD. Perhaps it was not the ideal time but, as people with children are very fond of pointing out, in variously patronising tones, there never is an ideal time.

In any case, it's the time we chose. I was twenty-six; he was thirty-one. We'd been together for six years already, more or less my entire adult life, a one-night stand that had, improbably, evolved into a partnership as intimate and banal as if we had set out to create it from the first. On the subject of children we were, always had been, agreed. There hadn't been one single moment of realisation that this was something we both wanted; we had, I think, taken each other's temperature over the years, hinted, questioned, until it became clear that we had the same kind of future in mind. But recently our hypothetical conversations had become subtly more concrete. For a year or so we'd been talking obliquely about it with something like intent – little conversations that always ended enthusiastically, but danced around the question of *when*, exactly.

Now it was early summer, the most promising time of year, the chill of spring well and truly gone, the days impossibly long. We'd walked to a pub by the river, where we sat drinking cider.

In a notebook we drew out possible timelines, determined that this was as good a time as any.

Why not now? When we had youth and optimism and ignorance all on our side: why not?

The prevailing cultural narrative around women's bodies, sex and childbearing had led me to believe – and I never questioned it – that this was a choice I could make, because, in spite of the best efforts of anti-abortionists, misogynists and all the rest, fundamentally, I had control of my own body. Of course that same narrative had taught me, too, that my body *needed* controlling; that it was always on the verge of disobeying orders, that its basic biological functions were at once necessary to life and necessary to hide, that I should mask any messiness, any leakiness: we must never show that we bleed or hurt or age, for we are only clocks, tick-tocking with mathematical precision towards and then away from some optimal reproductive moment.

For years I'd swallowed a pill at the same time every night, a simple solution; when, one evening, not long after that afternoon at the pub by the river, I took the last pill of the pack and threw next month's away, I was amazed by the ease with which I had transitioned into this next phase of life. When I woke up the next morning everything was coloured differently; the light was more hopeful, the sky was bluer, the famous golden stone of the city was warmer and more luminous than ever before. Everywhere were glimpses into a yearned-for future: the children careening down the street on their scooters, the mums clustered in the café, moving prams back and forth idly with one hand, sighing and soothing and sipping frothy coffees – even the green fecundity of an English summer, a thing so unlike the dry brown summers of my California childhood, a thing that couldn't help but make you *want*, and want, and want, and feel, soaked through by a sudden downpour on your way to get a sandwich for lunch, that anything and everything might be just on the point of happening.

We kept the decision close, like a secret, a precious thing. Only we knew about the pack of pills, the timelines in the notebook, the exciting irresponsibility of it all – we didn't even own a house, we didn't even have a savings account, we didn't even know when or if we'd get married, but we did know what we wanted, and we did know that it was our choice to have it now. An entitled attitude, yes; it had not yet occurred to me that simply to choose something like this did not give you a right to it. But the story I had in my head was simple and reinforced by things I'd read and seen and heard: that you decided to have a baby and then you had one. The decision was the thing that took the time and the work; now that we'd decided, we were more than halfway there.

I was not so much optimistic as oblivious. At a friend's birthday lunch, not long after throwing that pack of pills away, I sat with the knowledge of what we had decided, slightly apart, watching everyone getting afternoon-drunk. I happily declined another glass of wine, because I might be pregnant – I could be! It was possible. It was, even, likely.

I wasn't, of course, but how could I have known?

I awaited, each month, the fruits of our labour, which felt at this innocent point less like labour and more like fun, like something we were playing at. My body was a machine, built for exactly this purpose; it was only a matter of time.

Tick tock, tick tock.

At first every day, every hour, felt full of possibility. I made my daily pilgrimage to the pool and swam each morning with increased intensity, as if my body were gearing up for something, as if the water were not resisting my movements but aiding them, and I was so full of restless energy that after work, after dinner, after darkness had fallen, I couldn't sit still. I went for long walks round and round our neighbourhood, retracing my steps, passing the same lit-up houses and shuttered corner shops again and again. As I walked I let thoughts come that were not so much hopes as pleas: *this month. I can feel it.*

It's amazing what we can convince ourselves of, in hope or in fear.

A few months is no big deal. A few months is nothing. Doctors aren't interested in a few months. I wasn't even, at first, interested in a few months. A few months after I threw away next month's pack of pills it was still fun: a game whose resolution was already known, and so could be enjoyed without worry. Maybe this will be the last pint I have for a while, I would think, raising a glass to my lips – a notion somehow both cheering and chilling at the same time, since it spoke, in its own way, of the great truth that I hadn't yet acknowledged: that nothing can be known. *Maybe in a few days my life will look completely different. Maybe I won't need that box of tampons again for the better part of a year.*

Maybe I will.

A friend of mine tells me she went almost mad when she was trying to get pregnant, that she could hardly bear the wait, would buy each month – in spite of knowing better – a pile of pregnancy tests, and take them far too early, reading into every twinge, every slight shift of mood. It only went on for a few months, she says, but it felt interminable.

When she tells me this I think about the way I felt when I met her son for the first time, astounded by the fact that the last time I'd seen her, he simply hadn't *been*, at least not in the way he is now, a person, entirely separate from her, an externalisation of some secret effort. We had been in her sitting room, on the couch, the blue velvet one, eating toast slathered with butter and strawberry jam, watching Wimbledon, a hot day, she in a long tight jersey dress, belly enormous – and then the next time I saw her, there he was, her son, just like that, though of course for her it was anything but *just like that*.

It sounds stupid, but I'd never thought about birth as in any way miraculous before then; I'd never thought about the work that went into it, long before labour began; I'd never thought about the months that could feel like years, the weeks that could feel like months, the tricks that time plays on us all. I'd thought the narrative was uncomplicated, and linear, and inevitable.

One afternoon, a few months after we'd made our decision, I walked into town after lunch to buy a pregnancy test. Only a day late; unlike my friend I take an obsessively frugal approach to tests, tease the time for as long as I can bear. I won't take it today, I thought, I'll wait another day or two, but best to have it at the ready. Before I went into Boots I stopped at a shop across the street, drawing the errand out. It was very early autumn, mild, golden. They had coats on display, and idly I fingered them. One, Italian wool, dark grey, knee length, demanded to be tried on, though it was still warm out. I loved it. I looked in the mirror and thought I saw reflected back the version of myself that I have always wanted to be: someone put together, someone who wears simple, well-tailored clothes, who brushes her hair every morning and knows how to style it in a way that looks effortless but also deliberate; someone with a career, a purpose, a robust sense of self-worth, someone who is able, for example, to order a drink without prevaricating, to send an email without apologising, to walk into a crowded room at a party and not feel immediately and entirely at sea.

It was not too expensive, and I would need a new coat anyhow before winter set in, to replace my old moth-eaten duffle, but I quickly, decisively put it back on the rack.

I thought: *if the test is negative, I'll buy the coat.*

I wore it all autumn, all winter. What difference would it have made to buy it before I took the test? But it was magical thinking, a grasp at control. I remember all those pregnancy tests my friend took, when not a single one of them could alter the outcome, when not a single one of them could do anything but reflect her own unknowing back at her. All the walks, all the resolutions, all the bargains we strike, sometimes without even knowing we're striking them. The repetitions, the superstitions, that start to shape a life.

And then the start of a new month, and then another, and then the next.

★

That's how I got here – wherever *here* is. Here is now, and yesterday, and tomorrow. Here is the present tense. Here is in between and ongoing, waiting and wanting.

For some time now I have been on what I can only describe, although it doesn't feel quite accurate, since nothing is known, nothing is guaranteed, as the cusp of motherhood: almost motherhood, maybe-maybe-not motherhood. It's a place, sure as the swimming pool or the park or the pub on the corner of your road is a place – it's just not a very well defined one. Some people pass through it without even noticing; some people languish here for a little while, or a long while, held safe, held prisoner, by the walls of not-knowing – for as long as there is still a question mark, there is hope. In that sense we're all here, in one way or another: waiting for we-don't-know-what to happen, for love or success or a closure to grief, waiting for resolution, for a story to fold its arms around us, a neat before and after, a happy ending, or an ending, at least.

How to describe somewhere like that in language? If you think about it for too long it starts to shimmer and dissolve; its defining characteristic is always what it isn't. The best analogy I can think of for this is water, which has always, in some sense, eluded depiction, has always been something both essential to life and impossible to hold.

Of his famous paintings of swimming pools, the artist David Hockney once said: *I had become interested in the more general problem of painting the water, finding a way to do it. It is an interesting formal problem, really, apart from its subject matter; it is a formal problem to represent water, to describe water, because it can be anything.*

When I first read that I thought: *almost* and *maybe* can be anything, too. It is no coincidence that increasingly I find myself drawn to the swimming pool, to the edge of the water. Before I get in I like to stand, stretching my arms, adjusting and then readjusting my goggles, postponing the moment of immersion. I always check the clock on the wall before I drop into the water, so I know when I started. Submerged, heading for the other wall, I have no real sense of time, but that's not to say it isn't passing.

Tick tock, tick tock.

2

A Family Obsession

In the beginning it was the ocean that held me, not the pool. Some of my most visceral early memories are of the Pacific, glimpsed through living-room windows, experienced alternately as a source of comfort and fear: the security of being taken out past the waves by my father, the disorientation of being upturned by the roil of breakwater. I wore flipflops year-round, sand matted in my long hair, smelling of sunblock. I did not so much love the blue horizon as take it for granted. How else would I orient myself in the world?

My parents were living in Orange County when I was born, in an incongruously located trailer park on the edge of the affluent seaside city of Laguna Beach, just off the Pacific Coast Highway. So I come from the place that Ruscha has been so preoccupied with: southern California, with its parking lots, its pools, its dreams and cheap deceits. Sunshine in December, palm trees swaying, twelve-lane freeways, wildfires, mudslides. It's a place where things are often not quite what they seem, where a thin veneer of luxury has been spread over something wilder and harder, but in many ways it was an idyllic place to be a child; there were trips to Disneyland for my birthday, walks in the dusty backcountry, smooth, empty streets perfect for rollerblading or cycling – and always present, always at the edge of your consciousness, the wide, moody ocean.

Then, when I was eight years old, we moved to a cattle ranch up the coast, where my family had a parcel of land. They had bought it in the 1970s, when land was relatively cheap, intending someday to build a house there. The ranch was miles from anywhere, perched on the windswept ocean-edge of the state, separated from what I would, as a teenager, come to think of as 'civilisation' (a gas station, a grocery store) by a drive of at least forty minutes. The ranch was run as a co-operative; the land itself had been subdivided into parcels in 1971, on the proviso that individual owners could fence off a maximum of 2 per cent of their property, with the rest devoted to grazing. The result is a landscape that, relative to much of the rest of the state, seems frozen in time, or perhaps more accurately, exists outside of time – not only in terms of development but also in terms of the pace of life, the way that you are always to some extent at the mercy of bigger, baser things – sun, wind, rain – the way you might, driving to school, suddenly have to stop and wait for a herd of cattle to meander across the road, or pull over to marvel at the telltale spray from a whale's blowhole. This was not Ruscha's California. It was not really anyone's California, though perhaps Joan Didion comes closest, writing of the elemental pull of the West, its apparent indifference to human story: *The Pacific still trembles in its bowl. The great tectonic plates strain against each other while we sleep and wake. Rattlers in the dry grass.* It made you feel small, ultimately insignificant, or incidental at least: the snakes had made their home here too and it was your responsibility, not theirs, to keep an ear out for the threat of a rattle; the waves kept rolling in to shore regardless of whatever small drama had coloured your day.

It is not an easy place to explain, or indeed an easy place to live. More than 14,000 acres stretched along eight and a half miles of south-facing coastline, where the northern California ecosystem meets the southern California ecosystem. An in-between place: intertidal areas, migrating birds, unique flora and fauna. Looking westward is the Western Gate, what the Chumash called *Humqaq*, 'the raven comes', traditionally an opening into the celestial world, now home to a lighthouse, a stretch of railroad, an Air Force base beyond the point. Oil fields offshore produce tar that washes up on the beaches and sticks to feet, removed in my childhood with a vigorous scrubbing of WD-40 or, if it was particularly bad, white spirit. At night it is not quiet, like you might expect, but full of sound: coyotes howling, cattle braying on hillsides, owls, crickets, frogs, occasionally the guttural cry of a wildcat. My parents built their house so that it would function off the grid, powered by a set of solar panels, with water pumped from a well. Sometimes rains washed the road away in winter. Sometimes, if my dad was away working and we hadn't had any sunshine for a day or two, I would go outside and turn the generator on, come back inside smelling of wet sagebrush and petrol. I emptied the rat traps over the fence, where some scavenger or other would make quick work of the corpses. In summer I might step over a snake sunbathing on the deck, or sit watching lizards doing push-ups. I learned the contours of the hills by heart, by feel; I saw the sea every day, in every one of its innumerable moods.

I loved the ranch, I hated it. I felt its push and pull like a tide: the isolation, the beauty. Now I miss it, I dream of it. I left as soon as I could, at seventeen, off to university on the other side of the country. But I had, by then, begun to understand something fundamental about the way a place can mark you, the way it can settle under your skin, so that you are never really separate from it again, no matter where you are.

★

David Hockney, arriving in California for the first time in the early 1960s, was immediately gripped by the prevalence of pools: *as we flew in over Los Angeles,* he later remembered, *I looked down to see blue swimming pools all over.* I too, flying home, have often noticed this, as we dip towards the runway; all the little flashes of blue like punctuation marks in a landscape otherwise dominated by straight roads, strip malls, ticky-tacky houses that from a height, at least, do all look just the same. And when I see a pool I think immediately of *home*, wherever that is, wherever I am, and I want to sink into it, even just for a moment; I want to feel the water on my bare skin, the silk of the chlorine, the security of the embrace.

Pools have become a marker of home only retrospectively, however. When I actually lived in California I hardly gave them a thought – and perhaps that's the point, that you really only notice them from afar. As a child, pools were background noise; they were safe, decorative, convenient. They were for birthday parties and diving and holding your breath for as long as you could, for games – chicken fights, Marco Polo, sharks and minnows. Later they were for jumping into, in spandex shorts and sports bras, after a long, hot volleyball practice in the windowless school gym, in front of the wide-eyed boys. They were for my rich friends' parents to install and then ignore in the backyards of their sprawling new-build houses, houses that would never feel lived in, houses with too many rooms and too many empty cabinets.

They were always *there*, I just looked past them.

And then, when I was twenty, I moved away, to the other side of the world. To landlocked Oxford: as far from the sea, more or less, as you'll ever be in England. I had been interested from an early age in questions of geography: why did the place I was from seem to have such a hold over me, why did I feel the way I did, moved and steadied at the same time, looking out towards the oil rigs, lit up like burning ships on the horizon – and how, too, can another place pull you away, with even stronger force? I moved to Oxford to be with Alexander, who I had met by chance that summer, but also because sometimes, in the long evenings there, walking home, a blue veil falling over the terraced houses on the street where I was staying, a frail mist settling on my skin, the sound somewhere of bells ringing out, I had been overcome with something like mania, an almost physical need to be *here*, and nowhere else.

The question struggling to form in my mind had always been something like: *how does place shape us?* For a long time I thought that I could only ask this question of strong landscapes, storied cities. On top of a mountain, or folded into a walled medina, I might try to catch something of the answer on the wind: *who am I here? Where is the here in me?* But we spend most of our time elsewhere – in waiting rooms and supermarkets, kitchens and cubicles – and place, the geographer Yi-Fu Tuan reminds us, *exists at different scales*: at one end the favourite armchair, the body; at the other the country you come from, the whole earth. In other words, it is not only the mountains that make us, but also the small places, the in-between or invisible places – the narrow corridor of your commute to the office, the park you pass through every day, the room in which you lie awake at night, waiting for morning.

Over the years my view has narrowed. I did not intend it, but I stayed where I first stuck, in Oxford. I got a job, a dentist, a GP, a mobile phone contract. I bought a bicycle, learned the quickest routes through the city. Alexander and I acquired furniture: a bed, handed down from friends, a sofa, a set of ugly, practical oak bookcases. We rent a terraced house in a nice neighbourhood near a pub and a health food store and a halal butcher. Once there was the Pacific; now all I can see through my living-room window are the blue-painted window frames of the house across the street, and the red flash of the postman passing at midday, and our craggy old buddleia waving in a breeze. And most mornings, in this life, my other life, my everyday life, the life in which we are awaiting, not so very patiently anymore, the fruits of our labour, I wake up, get on my bike, and roll down the hill to the nearest indoor pool, where I swim laps, up and down, up and down.

*

It's something of a family obsession, water. I was steeped in watery stories from the start: my aunt, the elite diver who would likely have gone to the Olympics if the US hadn't boycotted the games in 1980; my grandfather, bodysurfing big waves in Newport Beach or swimming miles just for the hell of it; my dad, the swimmer, the water polo player, the lifelong surfer. One relative sends me an email: *As you may know, I often – and seriously – contend that I am a marine mammal. Simply cannot be me without the ocean.* My mother, on the other hand, a native New Yorker, never learned to swim, and has an equally intense but opposite reaction to the prospect of immersion. Comfort and fear, security and disorientation, expressions of the dual nature of water – *life-giving and murderous*, as Ivan Illich wrote. My mother's relationship to swimming, antithetical as it is, shaped me just as much as anyone else's, maybe more.

It's my grandmother, though, to whom I trace my love of the pool. She started swimming religiously – I can think of no better way to put it, though she is not a conventionally religious woman – in 1968, after an operation. The swimming was a thing to do to recuperate and rebuild strength after the operation; she had always liked being in the water, she said, growing up in Seal Beach, though she had to teach herself to do the strokes properly.

So it was circumstantial, really. But for some reason, or lots of reasons, it stuck. Maybe because by then her four children were old enough not to need constant care; her eldest son, my father, was eighteen, soon off to university. The others were not far behind, healthy, sporty, sociable kids growing up in an era and a household where independence was strongly encouraged. I picture time starting to pool in new places – in mornings or afternoons, in evenings, even. A quieter, or at least more self-sufficient, house.

Perhaps, too, it stuck because of that human instinct to replicate routine: we always seem to want to meet change with more of the same.

But this is conjecture. All I really know is that for as long as I can remember my grandmother has been a habitual swimmer.

She still drives the forty-five minutes from the ranch to a pool in nearby Santa Barbara a few times a week, unfailingly, unless she is ill, or rains have made the roads impassable. After her swim, she sits in the car and eats a packed lunch – a sandwich, macadamia nuts from the orchard, an orange, perhaps, if the season is right, or a white peach – before going to the grocery store to replenish supplies, and then driving home.

I started swimming regularly by accident, because of a minor running injury in my very early twenties. But really it was because of my grandmother: because there she was, all those years later, still wholly devoted to the ritual of going to the pool, getting in, going up and down, up and down. I was living in Oxford at this point, five thousand miles away from her pool, and my childhood view of the Pacific, but the first thing that popped into my head when my doctor suggested that I find an alternative to running, at least temporarily, was *water.*

On my way home from the GP surgery I stopped in at a JJB Sports, big, anonymous, windowless. It smelled of rubber and Lynx and mildew and no one offered to help me. I bought the cheapest swimsuit I could find without even trying it on, a pair of too-big goggles, a flimsy blue cap from which my hair seemed desperate, and destined, to escape. And later that afternoon I pushed open the doors to the pool nearest our house, which I had never visited before but had passed often and wondered about sometimes, and I entered.

★

If you visit a place, any place, often enough, it becomes interesting. This is how my obsession with the swimming pool began: at first so quietly I didn't even hear the hum, until it became a chorus I couldn't get out of my head, then a symphony that drowned everything else out. It happened by default, really, over a period of years; I simply went to the pool more often, more consistently, than I went anywhere else. I won't say it was love at first sight; it was a slow build. But I will say my interest in running waned. I found myself drifting instead down the road, to visit the pool as if it were a lover: my heartbeat raised in anticipation, my clothes left behind in a pile in a locker, my skin exposed. Sometimes after doing a few laps I would stand at the wall, ostensibly resting, for minutes on end, while everyone else kept chugging up and down. I was watching them, picking up tips. I tried to emulate the people who appeared most fluent. I tried to train myself to look like them – to look at home here. I went after work, or before, it didn't really matter, because there was always someone to learn from, or look at. Even when I wasn't at the pool I thought about my stroke. I watched YouTube videos on my laptop, read a book on technique my grandmother had sent me, stood in front of the mirror and moved my arms.

Eventually I bought myself a better swimsuit, a pair of goggles that didn't leak. Eventually I settled into a rhythm, in my own schedule, with my own stroke. Eventually I could not deny that I was a *swimmer,* that the pool was an important – *the* important – place in my life.

Early on, when I was still getting a feel for things, I booked a lesson with an instructor whose number was pinned to a notice-board at the pool. I had learned to swim so early in life I could remember it only in terms of vague impressions – sun, chlorine, shouts, splashes, goggles pressing rings around my eyes – but then I had taken the skill for granted, and it began to occur to me, as I sloshed up and down, that perhaps I needed to go back to the basics, to relearn good habits. The instructor watched me swim a few lengths. 'You're holding your breath underwater,' she told me eventually, and it's true, I was; I always waited until I turned my head to the side to quickly expel the old air and gulp some new air in. I should exhale steadily underwater, she told me: that way when I turned my head to breathe, I would have more time, and more capacity, to take in air.

It sounded simple enough, but to train yourself into a new way of breathing takes practice. To remind myself of what I should be doing I began to visualise the action as a blank space – the underwater exhalation – contained by a set of parentheses: the turn of the head to the side, the inhale. (   )

I was, at this time, making an attempt to be a freelance writer, but since my income from writing was virtually nil, I spent a few days a week working at a shop that sold novelty tea towels. The shop was fun, but no one came in; sometimes I would spend whole days without ever opening the till, without even saying more than 'hello' to a damp passer-by who had come in to shelter from the rain and who went away without even pretending to consider a purchase.

Apart from this and the pool I was alone a lot of the time – most of the time, maybe. Alexander had started a new job in London, waking up early to get a bus, coming home late, the structure of our evenings dependent on the whims of rush-hour traffic on the M40. After years of living too close in our small house in this small city we saw each other suddenly infrequent-ly, holding our bodies tightly together at night, spilling our frustrations and excitements out in a rush at the pub on Saturday evenings. When I was not at the shop I worked from home, or sometimes the library, where I would sit in obligatory silence, suppress my sneezes, and gaze out the window and watch all the people hurrying past on their bicycles or their mobile phones, people with somewhere to be. I had nowhere to be, really, but the pool. Maybe I was invisible, maybe when I spoke no one heard, but at the pool my body at least was irrefutable, a presence, displacing water, brushing up against other bodies on its journey up and down the lane.

★

Perhaps the most obvious defining characteristic of the swim-ming pool is its sameness, its uniform geometry. This has become, in a sense, a great comfort to me. I have come to think of it as something that has wrapped itself around me: a place of safety and security, a *container, a box of right angles*, as the sociologist Henning Eichberg has it, where *the peculiarities of the natural environment become smoothed out*. Eichberg did not write this uncritically, and it's possible for me to see how the containment, the chlorination, the imposition of rules and guidelines (no use of phones; no photography; no diving; no outside shoes beyond this point; no non-swimmers beyond this point), the insistence on selecting a lane to match your speed – slow, medium, fast – could be interpreted as oppressive. But what I want, as I drop into the water, push off from the wall and head towards the other end, is just this: clarity, containment, predictability, a straight clean line from A to B. What I crave, in this moment in time, is a landscape in which it is impossible to get lost, to stray too far, which is just what the container provides; you always know where you are in a pool, and if you don't, there's always something, or someone, to keep you in line.

But sometimes, still, I see something that unmoors me, something that doesn't fit, or fits differently. One day a spider scuttles along the wall in the changing room; on another day I find a cricket resting on a stack of communal kickboards. In spite of the no-outside-shoes-past-this-point rule mud is tracked into the changing rooms, mould blooms in the grouting of the shower, there is always the threat of the outside seeping in, or the inside spilling out, the threat of boundaries breached.

For example: once, as I arrived at the edge of the pool, ready for my daily submission, I saw a young woman with short black hair and a navy swimsuit emerge from the water with a nosebleed, bright red dripping onto the tiles, a shock of violent colour in the blue-and-white world. She held her head back, her hand to her nose, and she walked the length of the pool delicately, towards the changing room, vanishing from sight, and while I was doing my laps she vanished too from my mind.

But later, when I had come home, and settled at my desk with a pot of coffee, she returned, that image like a spot in my vision after staring at the sun – nature, as Yi-Fu Tuan writes, *not as an external environment but as our own body.*

If I think about it like that it becomes possible to see what I suppose I have always known, but had conveniently forgotten, that night when I threw out next month's pills: that the body is not machine but animal – and that we are as susceptible to the wilds of our own internal workings as to the sting of the wind on a summit or the bite of a spider.

★

When you swim, wrote the author and environmentalist Roger Deakin, *you feel your body for what it mostly is – water – and it begins to move with the water around it. No wonder we feel such sympathy for beached whales; we are beached at birth ourselves. To swim is to experience how it was before you were born.*

I recall his words as I slide below the surface one morning, about six months after Alexander and I made our decision to start trying for a baby: *how it was before you were born.* I push off from the wall and glide for a moment. I think *you* in the way that Deakin intended, as *me,* but I am also imagining another you, a future you, a you to whom I will someday say *before you were born,* a you to whom I am the before.

It occurs to me that I am only interested in all this now because I have a new sense of my own body: no longer abstract, no longer a thing to be taken for granted, no longer *the body,* in a sterile, academic sense, but *my* body, in a real, messy, frightening way that I haven't quite grasped yet. No longer wholly mine at all, in fact. I google things like *chlorine and conception* and *exercise in early pregnancy* and *should you do tumble turns if you might be pregnant?* Everyone has an opinion, although I never turn up any truly satisfactory answers; nothing ever seems to be as simple, when it comes to the body, my body, as yes or no, do or don't, can or can't, will or won't.

Before you were born. I mention all this in part as a way of saying that my relationship with water has always been based, in no small way, on geography and family history. But also because I think you can't write about the family you want – the family it's up to you to create – without writing, in some way, about the one you already have, the one you came from, the one about which there was no choice, no decision. Certainly I can't, just like I can't write about one kind of family obsession – which is to say, my desire, and so far, my failure, to start one – without writing about another: water, the pool, the *shifting mirror* (Illich again). When Alexander and I decided, definitively, to have a baby, I was of course looking, even if I didn't yet know it, for something that would help me make sense of the process. I found it in the pool, as I would have found it somewhere else had not the winds, the collective accident of birth, geography, upbringing, proximity, obsession, led me and kept me here.

But in a way, too, Deakin is right, it's deeper than that. It's the irrationality of it all, the inarticulacy of our own bodies. The wordlessness of the womb. Before I was born I was, as were we all, swimming in the soup of that *before*, lodged in the primordial place, the place of no speech, no memory. Everyone from Freud to the bin man, it seems, has a theory about water and wombs, about what a desire for submersion means. For Freud the symbolic meaning of a watery dream was to do with *fantasies concerning the intra-uterine life, the sojourn in the mother's womb, and the act of birth.* The Hungarian psychoanalyst Sándor Ferenczi, a colleague of Freud's, took the symbolism back even further, into evolutionary depths, suggesting that the desire to return to the womb was itself indicative of an even more primal desire to return to the sea from whence the human species came. What if, he posited, *the entire intrauterine existence of the higher mammals were only a replica of the type of existence which characterized that aboriginal piscine period?*

I don't know if I go in for all that stuff, but I'd be lying if I said the neatness of it didn't appeal: swimming as a kind of regressive comfort, a way to access again, if briefly, *the security and irresponsibility of the womb*, which is how Charles Sprawson describes it. Even to access, or grasp at, something before that, something beyond our collective memory. Every dip is like a taste you can almost but not quite describe; the only solution is to go again, and again, and hope that next time the words might come.

★

Words, words, words. When I swim laps they get lodged in my mind, phrases, snippets that I can't shake loose. My thoughts become something different to what they are on land; hardly formed, more like feelings, little kicks to the gut or the brain or some deeper part.

All the questions you can ask of a body. All the ways it can fail to respond; an unfamiliar sensation when in the past that body has always – more or less – bent to your whims: shrinking in response to decreased caloric intake, strengthening in response to increased exercise, changing or healing or behaving exactly *as expected*. And now what? It ignores the command; it carries on bleeding each month, it shows no sign of having heard the internal plea.

The mantra that becomes a game: *am I? Aren't I? Am I? Aren't I?* The rhythm that becomes a prison: *tick tock, tick tock.* The silence that becomes a sense: *something isn't working.* Everything deep, dark, drowned, felt but not known.

The problem with obsession, I'm learning, is that it doesn't clarify but distorts. It's a drug, not an answer. *A shifting mirror, a formal problem*: both ways of saying that the things we're most drawn to are often the things we cannot quite grasp, the things that in fact have no one shape but many. I want to understand my fixation on the pool; I want to understand my own body, and its apparent reticence in the face of what I am asking of it, which is essentially to make something entirely new out of almost nothing. But to do that I have to put words to places and processes that cannot or will not speak for themselves. To do that I have to think first about what things *are*, rather than what I want them to be, and that is harder than it sounds.

3

Before and After

There is *before* and there is *after*, and it is easy to feel that in a sense everything can be categorised as one or the other. Before you were born, and after. Before a major decision has been made, and after. Before a chance meeting that will change your life, and after.

Before I met Alexander I was a university student in Boston, majoring in political communication. I wore tight, low-slung bootcut jeans, cheap fitted blazers from H&M, had a side fringe and a fake ID which I used, with varying degrees of success, to try to get into bars with my friends who were twenty-one. My plan, which was a little hazy, was to graduate, get a paid internship while I studied for the LSATs, go to law school, move to Washington, D.C., and get a job. I did not actively want to be a lawyer, but I didn't see how it could hurt to have a law degree if I wanted to work in politics, especially since the acquisition of the degree would allow me to defer the decision of what kind of work, exactly, I actually wanted to do. I had begun my university career as an English major, but some pragmatic impulse had caused me to switch to politics halfway through my first year. What would I do with a degree in English? I'd always wanted to be a writer, but so did everyone else in my Intro to Fiction workshop, and I didn't see how there could be room on the shelves for all of us.

So in 2007, the year I turned twenty, I flew to Oxford for a six-week summer course in international relations. I was due to graduate that December and this was, I felt, my last chance to let loose before my Real Life began. The course was just an excuse, a jumping-off point; at the end of it I would buy a ticket to Berlin, where my best friend was studying German, and from there who knew? Budapest, Copenhagen, Prague, Vienna. Cities I knew only from books, from TV, from looking at maps and thinking the names sounded sophisticated and exciting, that I would like to be someone who could casually say, *Oh, when I was in Budapest . . .*

I had no ties to Boston; I had broken up with someone a few months earlier, and I was having casual sex with a friend from one of my classes, to whom I did not want to get too attached but knew I would if I stayed in the city for the summer. I worked as a temp for a company that provided catering staff for large events in the Greater Boston area, a job to which I was neither committed nor particularly well suited (at one charity fundraiser I dropped an entire tray of full champagne flutes and was so obviously flustered that a couple of the guests bent to their knees, in tuxes and ballgowns, to help me clear up); it was easy enough to hang up my stiff polyester suit, with its adjustable waistband and clip-on tie, and pack a suitcase.

On my first night in Oxford, the administrator of the international relations course took everyone to the pub, all twenty-odd young American undergraduates, with their jet lag and their shiny hair and their straight white teeth and their – *our* – uncharming innocence. At the pub I met Alexander, who was friends with the administrator. Standing outside in the summer crowd, drinking cheap fizzy cider and smoking Camel Lights, he and I got talking. We talked about where we were from, our families, the places we'd visited and wanted to visit, the books we loved, the books we were looking forward to reading. I told him I wanted to be a writer, even though I hadn't thought about this seriously in years, let alone said it out loud, and he did not laugh, or suggest this was an unlikely ambition. Maybe it was the cider, the electric summer air, but when I admitted my desire to write it did not sound as absurd as it had in the past; indeed, only a few weeks later I would give Alexander my laptop and let him see some stories I had written but not showed anyone, and he would read them late into the night, and I would fall comfortably asleep at his elbow, and in the morning I would feel neither embarrassed nor regretful.

We talked for so long that first night, and in such an insular way, that everyone we had been at the pub with – his friend, my fellow students – moved on, and we were still there. The pub closed and we drifted to a bar that was open late; the bar closed and we drifted down the High Street, hailed a taxi, took it to his house, which would someday be our house. At the time he rented it with a friend, an academic at the university, but she spent most nights at her boyfriend's place, and that evening we had the house to ourselves. Alexander's bedroom was sparsely furnished: a low futon bed, a blue cotton duvet cover, a small dresser, a hunting knife he'd brought back from Kenya hung on the wall. In the morning I had to be up early to get on a coach to go to Windsor. It was a bright, sparkling, early summer day, already warm – lucky, because all I had to wear were the clothes I'd had on the night before: a pair of flipflops, a flimsy black jersey skirt, a thin denim jacket. He walked me to the bus stop. On the back of an envelope that had once contained a gas bill he drew me a map, so that I would know where to get off the bus and how to find my way to the coach, and he wrote down his number. As the bus drew up he gave me his sunglasses, cheap Primark aviators that were too big for my face but which shaded my hungover eyes. Did we kiss? I think we must have, even though neither of us had brushed our teeth.

I did not have a mobile phone, at least not one on which I could dial the number written on the gas bill envelope (tucked in my suitcase was a little Motorola flip-phone which I would not turn on until I was safely back in the USA for fear of roaming charges). In Windsor I duly toured the castle with the other Americans, and then at lunchtime I peeled away from them and found a Carphone Warehouse, where I explained that I wanted the cheapest phone they sold. That evening, back in Oxford, I went out onto the street in Jericho where I was staying. It was another glorious evening, the light blueish-gold. Carefully I dialled the number, scrunched the envelope into my pocket. Perhaps he wouldn't answer; perhaps he would hang up as soon as he realised who it was; perhaps it wasn't even his real number, though something told me that he was not someone to whom it would occur to write down a fake number. The phone rang; I walked towards Walton Street, the main thoroughfare, past pubs and restaurants that were spilling onto the pavements. He answered. It was not awkward, or uncomfortable, though it could have been. I said I still had his sunglasses, if he would like them back. We agreed to meet the following evening at a pub in town, near where he worked. It was so simple it almost took my breath away; there was no coyness, no reticence, no sense that either of us was not genuinely interested in seeing the other again, no sense that games were being played.

After that we saw each other almost every day, mostly in pubs; when the pubs closed we would go back to his house and make gin and tonics and eat leftovers from the fridge: a chocolate cake, a roast chicken. The first time he invited me round for dinner I was anxious to seem like the kind of person to whom this was a habitual occurrence, even though the closest I'd ever come to being made dinner by a date was eating spaghetti with my ex-boyfriend and his housemates in a mouse-infested apartment near Fenway. Alexander was a good cook, which intimidated me, because I had somehow never really learned to cook, even though I'd been living away from home for more than three years now. At university I mostly made salads and pasta with jarred sauce for dinner, or else I microwaved veggie burger patties and ate them between slices of sourdough. I knew how to scramble eggs, how to make a balsamic vinaigrette, how to pit an avocado, but there ended my culinary abilities. He on the other hand could cook anything, or so it seemed: elaborate roasts, dauphinoise potatoes, tarte Tatin. That summer he taught me how to dice onions, how to poach an egg, how to make a crumble, which was not something I had ever eaten before, how to whip cream which had not come out of a spray can.

I remember the first night we spent together without having sex: we lay in bed, watching *High Society* on DVD; we fell asleep before the film ended. Maybe I already loved him then; certainly it was not long before we said it out loud, a few too many pints into an evening, embarrassed and then relieved. When my six-week course was up, instead of going to Berlin I simply moved in with him.

When we met, Alexander worked at a bookshop in town. He had thick brown hair, wore button-up linen shirts, jeans, Dunlop flashes, those Primark aviators. He carried a leather briefcase with him to the shop, containing a laptop, a book, and a small notebook in which he would sometimes make intricate little architectural sketches – a column, a door, a rooftop. Often, especially once my course was over, I would visit the bookshop while he was working; one day, sitting there, listening to the rain splashing down outside, we booked cheap flights to Fez. I had never been to Africa before. These are the kinds of things you can do, even if you're lucky, in only very rare moments of your life: meet a man, decide to move in with him, take an impulsive trip to Morocco. Would our relationship have developed differently, or at all, if there had been other constraints from the outset? If for example we were older, had established careers, caring responsibilities, mortgages, pensions, rhythms and routines that could not so easily be disrupted? It was not entirely straightforward – always at the back of our minds was the logistical question of how, when the summer ended, we would be able to be together, when we were not even citizens of the same country – but we had the incredible luxury of flexibility, of being able to fold our two lives into one, braid the strands together, each adapting according to the other's needs.

Of course it was not perfect, it was not effortless. We argued, even then, when there shouldn't have been much to argue about. I was jealous and possessive, perhaps because I was afraid there wouldn't otherwise be enough time: when I went back to Boston we would have an ocean between us, and then what? I compared myself unfavourably to the tall blonde colleague of his that he'd had a brief relationship with, even though I knew they had been unhappy together, even though I knew that he did not want to be with her; I bridled when he had obligations that did not or could not include me, even if they were banal in the extreme – a job interview, a catch-up with a friend he hadn't seen for years, dinner with his family. I felt at times that I had been swallowed up by our love, as if there were nothing else in the world but *us*, or at least nothing else I cared about. I was on antidepressants that, although I didn't know it at the time, reacted badly with alcohol, and sometimes when I drank too much I became despondent, recklessly sad or angry about nothing in particular. Alexander, meanwhile, had his own foibles: an irresponsibility about money that caused us both stress; an intense, infuriating desire to please everyone all the time, which sometimes – often – meant that in fact he instead let everyone down. As much as we loved each other it would have been easy enough, I suppose, at the end of the summer, to simply go our separate ways.

Back in Boston, though, I could not imagine a future without him. We chatted over Skype every couple of days; my laptop didn't have video capability, so he couldn't see me, but I could see him, and the achingly familiar house: the kitchen where one night, drunk, I had sat on the black and white tiled floor wearing nothing but a pair of pants, one of Alexander's shirts, and the paper hat from a Christmas cracker that I'd found in a cupboard, eating a sandwich; the sunny bedroom in which I had woken up every morning for almost the entire duration of our relationship; the overgrown garden, now shedding some of its summer green, paling at the edges.

I missed him – the way he called me 'darling' without a trace of irony or affectedness, the smell of him, the substance of him – in a way that hurt. I missed the city itself, everything I felt it held: possibility, unknown promise. I wanted to be there, not here. I had, I realised, without really meaning to, made a definitive choice, a commitment, to another person, to a future together. I researched visas, found that I could apply for a six-month work permit, sent in my completed forms and a $500 processing fee. In the meantime I had a few months of classes left, a thesis to write, but I cared very little about my studies at this point. I was just killing time.

At the end of the semester, Alexander flew out to Boston to help me pack up my things. I sold all my furniture, such as it was – a plastic kitchen table and two folding chairs, a futon bed and mattress, a large wooden desk and a stool – to the daughter of a colleague of my father's who had just moved to Boston. I used the money I made from the sale of the furniture to ship every book I owned to England: $900 worth of boxes, which we spent an afternoon lugging to the post office and standing in line, days before Christmas, to post.

Weeks later, when the boxes finally made it to Oxford, we took my books and mixed them with his on the shelves. An almost reckless act of faith so early on in a relationship: what's mine is yours.

★

I think about this a lot these days – the way your life cleaves invisibly, irrevocably, the moment you make a decision, the moment you make a commitment. *Before, after*: but what of the space between the two words, the comma, the pause, the breath taken? What if you get stuck there? What is that landscape, that empty sea?

Before, we sat cross-legged on the kitchen floor, drinking gin and eating chocolate cake. We stayed out late every night, talking, listening. Sometimes it seemed like we were always drunk, because the evenings were so long, so frequent. We acted impulsively, did not take our jobs seriously, invited friends round for elaborate Sunday lunches that would go on until the early hours of Monday morning, booked trips we couldn't really afford to take, made no plans or reservations until we got there. We thought about the future only in very limited terms: this month, next month, then who knows. We had the great privilege, which perhaps we did not recognise at the time, to do this, and we eluded responsibility for a very long time, longer than we should have. We pushed it away again and again. But now it seems like when we want it, when we've gone out seeking it, even though we are calling for it, it will not come.

4

An Invisible Threshold

Writers on swimming are fond of the threshold metaphor: water as boundary between worlds, as crossing-place. *Leaving behind the land,* Roger Deakin writes, *you go through the looking-glass surface and enter a new world.* What lies beyond the looking-glass surface, though, is harder to describe; like water itself it is slippery, difficult to pin down with language. There's something drug-like about it, tempting, dangerous maybe; Charles Sprawson wrote that, like opium, swimming *can cause a sense of detachment from ordinary life.* Maybe this is so: for a moment, taking the plunge into pond or pool, we become someone else, something else. The swimmer is at once contained in their own world – the world of self, of thought, of bodily awareness – and transported elsewhere, nowhere, everywhere – as if to swim laps were a form of everyday escapism, in the vein of Tuan, who asks: *But what if the 'place' one wishes to escape from is one's own body? Can one take flight from one's own corporeal wrapping?*

To swim is, in some sense, to take flight: in the pool, we are lighter, we are no longer sure which way is up, we are no longer, biologically at least, at home, and so we are also somehow cheating or tricking our own physiology. No one in my lane cares whether I can or can't conceive. What the water knows it keeps to itself. Wherever I am in my cycle it takes me roughly the same amount of time to swim 400 metres. My body, I remember here, has substance and significance beyond its reproductive function. I feel a snap of pain as my hand hits the plastic lane line; I pause at the wall, breathing hard, chest rising and falling; I take a moment, when I have the lane to myself, to float on my back, kicking gently, staring at the ceiling.

But what does this do to us when we come out, grounded again, landbound, and find ourselves stuck still in our everyday lives, heavy animals, bound by our corporeal wrapping, with all the demands of the day ahead of us? I have never found this an easy transition, but I notice it more now than ever, as if there's a crack, a lag, as if I am in fact becoming two bodies.

The laps are one thing; the safe thing. After the laps, outside the pool, is something else.

★

I have crossed an invisible threshold. A few months was nothing to be concerned about; almost a year is something else, is edging towards anomaly. I am still young, but I am slipping out of, or into, statistics: we are not among the 20 per cent of couples I read about in one article who will conceive in the first month, then not among the 72 per cent of couples who will conceive in the first six months, then not among the 84 per cent of couples who will conceive in the first year. I fixate on these numbers, even though the article cites no sources, cannot be considered reliable; they indicate to me that I am unusual, an exception, and not in a good way. When I go hunting for more definitive statistics about the likelihood of conception I discover that they are difficult – almost impossible – to find: there are too many complicating factors, like age, to allow for a clear-cut consensus. Perhaps this should be encouraging, but to me it only underlines the magnitude of my failure: that I cannot get even this most basic, essential biological process right, that by most measures I am an outlier.

Doctors are mildly interested in the fact that I am not yet pregnant – mildly because of my relative youth; interested because there is no obvious reason that a woman of twenty-seven, otherwise healthy, with no clear impediment, should be having such trouble conceiving. My blood is taken again and again, in alarming quantities, sometimes at various specific points during my cycle: between days two and five, to check my levels of follicle-stimulating hormone; on day twenty-one, to check for evidence of ovulation. To some extent the precision of these tests is futile in the face of the messy biological reality of having a body; it assumes a textbook twenty-eight-day menstrual cycle, but like many women, my cycle varies by a few days from month to month, and so the day twenty-one test may actually need to take place, for example, on day twenty-five. It takes a few months to nail the right day, and in the end, nothing in particular can be determined. There is evidence of ovulation; my thyroid function is healthy; I do not have any STIs; all the test results, in other words, are normal. An ultrasound reveals an unusually shaped uterus – *bicornuate*, heart-shaped – but this, the doctors agree, is in itself not likely to impede conception, though it might have implications later. The ultrasound also indicates that I might, but don't necessarily, have polycystic ovary syndrome – a common and varyingly impactful condition that can, but doesn't necessarily, affect fertility. It's hard to say for sure, my GP shrugs, how much any of this has to do with anything else.

I don't know whether to be soothed or alarmed by the equivocation, all these *coulds, mights, maybes, probablies*, these *we just don't knows*. How can you not know? I want to shout at every doctor who shrugs at me – but I'm equally frightened, if I'm honest, of an unequivocal answer, a *definitely this*, a prescription, a path, a trap, a *never*. So I stay here, adrift in the land of almost, of maybe, and part of me is not entirely unhappy to be here, part of me is in fact afraid of asking the right questions, even while I'm drowning in the silence of my own body. *Speak*, I think to it, late at night, but it says nothing, or nothing that I can translate.

★

In July, over a year after we made our decision, we attend the wedding of some close friends of ours. They have hired a swanky hotel in the Cotswolds for the occasion. The weather is perfect: fair skies, hardly a breeze, so that they can be married outside, under an archway, on an emerald lawn into which the spikes of my pale blue heels keep sinking. The bride wears shiny gold brogues with her vintage dress; their toddler son attends in waistcoat and bow tie. At dinner I realise that the woman I am seated next to is not drinking because of the bump half-hidden beneath the drape of the trapeze dress she is wearing. I realise, too, that I have forgotten to regulate my own intake of alcohol, even though my period is due in a few days, even though I *might* be pregnant, I could be, it's possible, but, I find myself thinking, increasingly unlikely. I am tipsy from too much champagne sipped in sunshine; I reach across the table, pour myself a very full glass of red to see me through the speeches. I feel a little ugly, a little ragged – envious of the woman in the trapeze dress, envious of the bride and groom and their handsome little son in his waistcoat and bow tie, furious at myself for letting go of the reins of self-control, for giving in to doubt – but on the other hand here I am, all dressed up, surrounded by friends, and wouldn't it be a shame if I didn't let myself enjoy it? I have no energy left, in this moment, to maintain hope while also holding the possibility of disappointment close.

The truth is that I have stopped treating every month like it's the last month of my old life, have stopped obsessively restricting my consumption of wine at birthdays and weddings and lunches and dinners, because that's no way to live, as if always on the edge of something, as if always just about to leave, like arriving at a party and not taking your coat off even though the room is full of bodies and the radiators are turned all the way up.

But I have not stopped keeping track, even if obliquely, of where we are, have not stopped keeping score, have not, in other words, given up, even if I'm running low on optimism. Sex is fraught. Everything is fraught, in its own way. Even the desire itself for a child, once a purely hopeful thing, is tainted. Do we deserve this? Want it really, or enough? Am I in fact somehow standing in my own way; is my reproductive system trying to tell me something that my head and my heart won't hear? Are we good enough, are we in love enough, are we people for whom others will be happy when or if we make the announcement? Or is the universe trying to say that we will be bad parents, that we are not suited to making this journey, that we are not as ready to embark as we thought we were? A niggle of doubt about the foundations on which our relationship is built crows for attention: what are they really? Will they hold? We were fine when it was all cider and sunshine and abstract timelines in a notebook, but what if we are not up to the challenge of the tangible reality?

One day, on the early-morning bus into London for a meeting with my PhD supervisor, exhausted, the shadow of a last-orders-at-the-bar-induced headache behind my eyes, I find myself actually grateful not to have the complication of childcare, of physical and emotional dependency, of someone else, someone essentially helpless without me. I am broke, my erratic freelance income never seems to arrive when most needed, the small stipend I received at the start of my PhD has long since been spent, the edges of the future are fuzzy at best: what good would I be to a child? What good, come to that, would a child be to me? A terrible thought, but not an illogical one. I slump against the window, watch the familiar landmarks slide past – the self-storage centres, the mattress superstores, the Hoover Building, Park Royal Station. As we stop-and-start along the Westway, I can see into the glittering interiors of the high-rise offices near Paddington. Someone is climbing a flight of steps, holding a white mug. Someone is taking a jacket off. Lots of people are sitting at desks, pulling their chairs in, moving stacks of papers, leaning towards the blue glow of their screens, holding phones to their ears. One woman is standing at a photocopier, waiting while page after page is reproduced, the tray still filling as the bus jolts forward and away. I envy her, though I couldn't quite say why: is it the simplicity of her task, the blind purposefulness of it? Yes, I think, she's useful. She is serving a function. Someone somewhere is relying on her to do this job, and she will not disappoint them.

That evening Alexander and I have a fight about who let the milk run out, then about what to eat for dinner, then about nothing in particular, but it feels good to fight.

We fight often, these days. We fight about money. We fight about work – mine, his. I am angry because his employer is making unreasonable demands of him, his time; what I am trying to say is that I think he's being undervalued, that I think he's undervaluing himself, that I will fight his corner even if he won't, but it comes out wrong, like an accusation, like a complaint. He not infrequently comes home from work late, a little drunk, and gets up very early, a little hungover, to go back into London. We fight about that, too, but only half-heartedly; at the end of the day we are too tired for blame, really, can both see the other's point of view before it has even been articulated.

This did not come from nowhere. We have always had fights about milk and money and nothing in particular, are both prone to talking – shouting – our way through something, in a *better out than in* kind of way, and then to making up, moving on, without much fuss. But what is different now is the withholding, the undertones, everything charged by the things we aren't saying, the things we won't admit.

If I would only say *I'm scared*, or he would only say it. But of course neither of us does, or perhaps neither of us can, and so we go on flailing silently and stubbornly in this new territory, *through the looking-glass surface*, where everything is murky and grey.

5

The Trick

The trick, some people say, trying to be helpful, is simply to stop wanting it: *my wife and I had all but given up when . . .* Even my GP, who I have always appreciated for his irreverent, no-nonsense attitude, slides into uncharacteristic sentimentality and tells me a version of this story, a couple he'd been seeing for years. He was in the process of referring them for IVF when . . .

But how to trick yourself into not wanting something you want? I start to feel a rift opening up between myself and my body; how can I convince it, I wonder stupidly, that, in fact, I don't care whether it conceives or not?

But what if the 'place' one wishes to escape from is one's own body? What indeed? What then?

6

An Escape, Almost

At the start of the year, about six months after our decision, I joined a triathlon club. I have no intention of doing a triathlon – or maybe I do – but I like having other people to swim with. It was to begin with just a New Year's resolution: to do something *physical*, by which I meant something more taxing than my gentle daily swims, something more punishing. It did not seem enough, anymore, to adhere to my old routine; my old routine was not working. I wanted something new, some way to test the capabilities and limitations of my body, some proof of my own youth and vitality. And I wanted it to hurt a little, because it felt as if I deserved that; if my body would not obey in one arena, then by force I would master it in another.

Before joining the club I attended a trial swim session. I closed my laptop early one evening and cycled across town, stammered my way through an introduction, sure I'd be the odd one out, but everyone was welcoming. I was not made a fool of; I was not out of place. A pool is a pool, after all, and while I don't know much, I do at least know how to go up and down a lane and not crash into anybody else.

It makes me a nicer person – or a person, at least, which is a start. To have a thing. To have a thing that forces human contact, that requires me to situate myself, even briefly, in relation to others. A thing that encourages me to *use* my body.

So now, on Mondays and Wednesdays and sometimes Fridays, I make my way to various pools around the city and I spend an hour, or sometimes an hour and a half, nearly naked with a bunch of nearly strangers: people I know by name and by swimming speed and by not much else. We do drills, time trials, once or twice a relay race. There is a sense of camaraderie tinged with competitive intent; everyone, of course, wants to be the fastest person in their lane, everyone is really there for their own personal gain, their own secret reasons. This is very simple, very easy for me to understand: that the more I swim, the more I practise, the better, the stronger, I will become.

One night I tell one of the coaches that my one goal, my only goal, is to get faster. He breaks it down for me: I need to think about shaving milliseconds off the time it takes me to swim 25 metres, not minutes off the time it takes me to swim 400. Do it slowly, incrementally.

He's right, of course, though at the time I am disappointed that there isn't a magic fix.

One of the pools that the club uses is a few miles out of town, and so on Wednesday evenings I get a lift with Alan, who lives around the corner from me. He's married, balding, in his forties, an ex-rower with, I suspect from the way he talks about the Ironman he's training for, a penchant for a particular kind of physical punishment that now, in his softer years, is harder to come by except in extremes. We swim in the same lane, at roughly the same speed, and although we have otherwise little in common, our conversation in the car is easy, comfortable. I start to look forward to it, as if it's an integral part of my Wednesday workout: the walk to his house, the knock on the door, the casual luxury of the old BMW estate. I realise that it's because I can control, almost entirely, what he knows about me, and so, to an extent, what he thinks about me. I can be someone who swims hard, who is – maybe, although I am very cagey about this – *in training* for something. Someone, in short, who is in control.

One evening, on the way home, he mentions a friend of his who he bumped into recently, who he used to go running with; 'but she's pregnant now, of course,' he says, disparagingly, and I find myself laughing along, and I see that I have done a good job of presenting a particular version of myself, that I have split myself successfully into two – or else that my desires are somehow less clear-cut than they used to be, that everything is folding in on itself. Too late, much too late, it occurs to me to wonder if he and his wife have no children by choice or by circumstance, or if perhaps I am not as opaque as I think.

I know that I am at the pool a lot. One Wednesday evening, I spend 200 metres thinking solely about what an odd way this is to spend a Wednesday evening. I think: I'm an adult. I'm not compelled to do this. It serves no purpose. I could be catching up with a friend, or lying on the couch, watching a crime drama, or having sex, or reading a book. But it's an escape, almost: the moments when it becomes hard to focus on anything other than the weariness, the need to carry on, the water churned up, the sheer relief of not thinking too much, except to count the laps, except to remind myself not to turn my head so far when I breathe. It's imperfect, as a mechanism; my mind does drift towards this or that, towards the sharp little misgivings that sing loudest into silence, but eventually, usually, it comes up against the barrier of my own physical exertion, hits the wall of the pool and stills, at least for a time.

The architectural historian Thomas van Leeuwen wrote: *While the pool allows, even invites, intellectual wanderings, at the same time it prevents the wanderer from losing his way . . . The container encloses but also retains, holds together, and keeps from spilling.*

There is less room for doubt here. If I can only be kept from spilling, held together—

I am still playing a game, though, hedging my bets. When the other members of the club ask me what races I've entered I shrug, too embarrassed to admit that while I am ostensibly in training, I'm not in training for anything in particular; that while I am swimming and running most days I am also still hoping, each month, for a different and more definitive kind of physical transformation. *If I'm not pregnant next month I'll sign up for a triathlon*, I think. I'm not, but I don't: a funny sort of stasis. I just keep going up and down the lane each week. In the meantime, I think. Mean time.

7

In Parenthesis

In a novel, I once read this:

If there were even the slightest chance, Ester would think of nothing else and live in parenthesis until that day arrived.

I think about this line a lot. About what parentheses signify, what they contain. A blank space, a possibility. But also something like an afterthought, an aside. They are made to interrupt, but gently, the softness of their curved shape like a half-formed thought. What they hold is an indulgence, not a necessity.

Somewhere in the house I grew up in, there is a photograph of my mother and a close friend. They are both about eight months pregnant, my mother with me, her friend with her daughter, standing back to back with bellies bared. 'Bookends', someone has scribbled on the back of the photo. But these days I can only see parentheses, that long, empty exhalation: ( )

If only, I sometimes think, I had known how long I myself would be living in parenthesis – but then again, what good would knowing do?

8

A Decision in the Mind

It would be dishonest, wouldn't it, to imply that once a decision has been taken there can be no doubts. That a decision is concrete, or carries any weight at all in the republic of the body. *A decision in the mind is pretty small,* Sheila Heti writes of the choice to have children. *It doesn't make babies.*

When we sat by the river, over a year ago now, and ordered another two bottles of sweet cloudy cider, and poured them into glasses sticky with the anticipation of summer, we were enacting a sort of ritual of decision-making, pretending to have already moved into a new place, pretending that that's all it takes. We weren't as stupid as perhaps I have implied, though we were certainly more naïve than we are now. We knew there was a chance of things not going to plan, we knew there were factors outside our control, we knew that for some people, for many people, it isn't as simple as *a decision in the mind.* When I first met Alexander, he told me that he'd had a brother and sister who had died – twins – born premature. He was seven at the time, remembers holding them at the hospital, knowing he would never hold them again. Before he was born, his mother had been told she couldn't have children, so he was a surprise, and then his parents laboured for nine years to have another child, or children, until his brothers – more twins – were born and lived.

A lie, then, or at least a misremembrance, to say we had no warning, no doubts, no alternatives to the simplest story, the

45

one we're not-quite-told, that all it takes is a conviction, a choice.

What we didn't know, couldn't know, was what it would *feel like*. What it would make us think, and say, and do, to each other, to ourselves. That some of these would be terrible things, but not all of them, not even most of them.

Somewhere along the way, we decide to get married. Not because of but in spite of. It could so easily have gone the other way. All the moments in a relationship where a different word could have been said, a different decision made, a different tone of voice used. Nothing holding us together but habit, and inertia. And love, of course, but love is a funny thing, that can sometimes feel like hate, or apathy, or nothing at all. It's true that the longer you live with someone the harder it becomes to extricate *me* from *you*; you lose track of whose copy of *Les Grand Meaulnes* that is, whose spatula, whose towels, whose toothbrush, whose friends, everything entering the ambiguous realm of *us*, *ours*. But somewhere I read that a marriage, or a partnership, is just an ongoing process of choosing and then choosing again to stay put; to enter into such a contract, then, is not a single decision but an unending series of them. I have a friend who left her fiancé a few months before they were due to get married. There was no one factor, no great rift: she simply woke up one morning with a clear head and an urgent desire not to go any further down that path, an utter lack of curiosity about where it led. To choose to go further down the path can be the same – no grand gesture, because a life together is a grand enough gesture, in its own way; no tipping point; just a simple capitulation to more of the same.

And so one bright, blustery Saturday afternoon we walk into town, have a couple of stiff drinks at a hotel bar, go across the street to a jeweller and buy a very small diamond ring. *It's about time*, people say, when we tell them, as if they have known all along something that we have only just learned. We were not actively avoiding it – we had I think always intended to get married, at some point – but I remember that when we sat by the river and said *why not now?* we also agreed that we were happy to have children before we had a wedding, that there was, in a way, less urgency about marriage, by which I guess really we meant it was something we could control, something we could slot in when it fit. I pictured, charmingly, a son or a daughter toddling through the throngs, lifted onto shoulders for photographs, disrupting the ceremony with a laugh or a cry, swept away at an appropriate hour by doting grandparents. But these are other people's memories; they belong elsewhere.

For a while we are reluctant to set a date, to do anything concrete about it, although neither of us will admit to the other why exactly this is. At the back of my mind is still the unknown: the maybe, almost, the possibility, the green promise of summer still hanging on the air.

But life has to go on, doesn't it? If we hold our breath forever, we'll just be holding our breath forever.

Two

A Wild Place

2014

I

In Control

During the 2012 Olympics I became obsessed with watching the swimming on TV. Because the Olympics were being held in London, I could watch every event in real time: the heats in the morning, the important semi-finals and finals in the evenings. At first I attempted to ration my consumption, telling myself that after, say, two heats I would get back to work – but eventually I could not honestly claim that I was doing anything other than watching hours of Olympic coverage each day.

If you've ever watched competitive swimming, you will know that, while it can be exciting, particularly in the last breathless milliseconds when outcomes are decided, in essence it's a predictable, repetitive sport, played out in the tame amphitheatre of the pool. Not like a football match, for example, where anything might happen in the interaction between two teams, between so many teammates, where a crack of thunder and a sudden downpour might change the whole tenor of the contest. Most of the races don't last very long, a few minutes maybe, under twenty-five seconds for a fifty-metre sprint; you might spend more time watching the swimmers preparing to race, unzipping sweatshirts, adjusting hats and goggles, swinging their arms, than actually racing. But I loved the discipline of it, of the bodies in particular. Swimming is a sport where the body is undeniably *on show*, the athletes barely clothed, in suits tight as skin, and these most elite bodies had been trained and honed to such an extent that they made everything they did look somehow both impossible – for the rest of us, at least – and easy. They had been *made*, quite literally, for this.

Sometimes, in interviews or profiles, you might get a glimpse of what the swimmers' lives were like: multiple training sessions a day, up and down, up and down a pool, for thousands upon thousands of metres. They were on their own a lot of the time, even if they trained with other people, because the underwater nature of their sport precluded most conversation. It was hard, it was boring, but it was the only way. (I remember my dad describing swim practices at his high school in the 1960s; 10,000 yards in an under-heated pool, the slog of it, the meanness of the coaches, the wild hunger of the swimmers afterward, and this was only for the sake of small-scale, regional competition.) The athletes talked a lot about *pushing themselves*. One anecdote in particular has always stuck with me: the young medal-hopeful Hannah Miley describing how one day, during a training session, she punched a wall. *I thought 'I just want some other part of my body to hurt',* she told an interviewer. *All I wanted to do was to take the skin off my knuckles so that the chlorine would really sting. I knew if that happened, then when I started swimming again I would think about the stinging rather than the real pain.*

Commentators, I've noticed, often talk about how much competitors *want it*: wanting it being, in commentator parlance, a signifier not only of how much someone has given up but also how much they deserve to get in return, though it doesn't always pan out that way. I was compulsively interested in the single-mindedness required to push past not just basic human needs and desires – for sleep, for rest, for *just one more* at your local on a Friday evening – but pain itself. To, in fact, have a hierarchy of pains, to play them off each other, all in service of a single unlikely goal. I was also interested in the notion of sacrifice: swimmers sacrificing 'normal' relationships, giving themselves up completely to the competition; parents sacrificing time, money, their own desires or pleasures. Everything done on a hope, of course. (Miley never did get her Olympic medal, though she came close.)

So I would sit at home on a Tuesday morning with my laptop open, watching some fifteen-year-old whiz-kid breaking a world record, and I would think how simple it must be to have something so concrete to work towards: an end goal, a singular achievement, a step up to a podium, a medal hung round a neck. There is something pure and admirable about this, or at least about the approach, something deliciously counter to the ambiguity that characterises so much of ordinary life. *After twenty years I still search for the dumb focus I had as a competitive swimmer,* the artist Leanne Shapton writes. *After a hundred workouts I might be faster,* she says, whereas when it comes to her work, her art practice: *After a hundred pages, a hundred sketchbooks, when will it feel right?*

Of course the conclusiveness, the neatness, of competitive sport is part of what makes it so compelling: a winner and a loser, this person objectively faster than that one, and therefore, for the purpose of the competition, *better.* Most of life isn't like this. At work, in relationships, we have to guess, feel our way through. We don't get the satisfaction of a podium, the din of a supportive crowd, a newspaper headline – but then again, neither do most athletes.

And, sometimes, a race would be so close that it all seemed arbitrary. If two contestants are really so equally matched, what's the deciding factor? Not skill, or strength, or speed, but something else, something that can't be worked for, or controlled, not even after years of practice.

★

Where I grew up there was always risk. Wherever you built, wherever you staked a claim, something at some point would come along to remind you of the fragility of that claim: a fire, a flood, a rattlesnake stretched across a doorway. California is like that, *a society built on quicksand,* as the writer Pico Iyer once put it, but the ranch, because it was relatively remote, relatively undeveloped, seemed to exaggerate this tendency towards chaos. It had an uncanny beauty that gripped you and held you tight, all the more so for the way it seemed always about to slip out of anyone's control. My memories of it are more like feelings, flashes of impression – cold Pacific blue, the smell of hot dust, a coyote howling, a wind, a fog, a big black cow, a sea of dry grass.

I was often afraid of the water, or wary at least. It's one thing to grow up with a love of the ocean, and to know enough to respect it; another thing, though, to be a naturally fearful child surrounded always by threat. Nothing was safe, and if you dwelled on it too long it became impossible: a mountain lion *might* be lurking in the trees, a snake *might* be hidden in the grass, the smoke wafting on August air *might* presage disaster. A wave rolling at you in that wide expanse might take you with it, and I was slow to learn to trust, too often dragging my heels in the sand, lurking in the shallows, waiting for a calm still day, the kind the surfers all eschewed, when I could paddle an old foam board out to the kelp bed and anchor myself there for a while, watching the shore.

When I discovered the swimming pool, then, I think I also discovered what *control* feels like. The neatness of my Oxford life, with its ordered streets and terraced houses, gave me a sense of safety. Wildlife was a cartoon novelty: a fox poised in the middle of the road at midnight, a magpie, a cat in the garden, stalking a fly. If I went out into the dark, as I sometimes did, to feel the rough city air on my skin, the shadows moving at the edge of my vision were only other night-walkers, swaying drunk or striding home. When I slid below the surface of my favourite lane at the pool I was going up against nothing more or less than my own ability, my own tautness and discipline.

I have begun recently to think of swimming at the pool as a form of *pure* swimming. By which I mean the only kind of swimming I can do that lets me get a measure of myself: how fast I am, how efficient my stroke is, what improvements I've made. It's an addiction, of sorts, to the idea of physical progress, which is something I cannot gauge in wilder waters, where wind or waves might throw me off course.

Sometimes, when I am doing something very banal – slicing an onion, walking to the bus stop, pruning a rose – I wake up for a moment to the fact of my body *as* me, the plain physical pleasure in a tear forming, a step taken, a thorn biting. But most of the time, and I don't think I'm alone in this, I think only of the function of my body, the mechanics and measurements of it, what it can *do*. Or can't do, or won't do.

It being an object somehow both of and outside myself.

In exercise, the author Mark Greif writes, *one gets a sense of the body as a collection of numbers representing capabilities.* Greif points out that one of the only other places where numbers hold this kind of importance in relation to the body is at the doctor's office or the hospital: height, weight, blood pressure, body fat, cholesterol levels, blood test results, scans. But whereas at the doctor's office, numbers are assigned to us seemingly without our control or consent, at the gym or the pool, numbers become something we believe we can change. Any failure to do so is a failure of self-control and resolve, not biology.

The simple fact of the matter is that I have started to rely on swimming as a kind of measure of my success as a body. 'I think you might be in the wrong lane,' a coach at one of the triathlon club sessions says one evening, because I'm having a good day, and I'm faster than everyone else in the lane. *Progress,* I think smugly, though I demur out loud – 'oh, no, just a fluke.' But the next week I'm not the fastest, and the next lane up seems like a pipe dream. *Work harder,* I think in the lucid moments between sets, as if I can will myself stronger, better, which it seems I can. In fact swimming on its own is not enough: I take longer and longer runs, start training at the track once a week, sign up for a half-marathon. I'm no longer under any illusion that it's camaraderie or fun or external validation I'm after. I'm only doing it so that when I look at myself in the mirror I see a body I like the look of, a body that's disciplined, in control. A body, in other words, that does what it's told.

The philosopher Susan Bordo wrote: *the firm, developed body has become a symbol of correct* attitude; *it means that one 'cares' about oneself and how one appears to others, suggesting willpower, energy, control over infantile impulse, the ability to 'shape your life'.*

Well, I want to shape my life. I am shaping my life. The shape of my life is muscular shoulders and legs that can carry me for miles. If I can't control my womb, if my *dumb focus* on my reproductive ability is not getting me anywhere, then at least, I think, at the very least, I can control the rest of myself.

2

A Beginning and an End

In September, well over a year after we first made the decision to start trying for a baby, we go to Dartmouth for a week with Alexander's parents. They have rented a holiday cottage at the mouth of the river and invited us along; we are broke, and quick to seize the opportunity to get away from the city, to spend some time at the edge of the land, looking out towards the sea. For Alexander it is a sentimental trip: his family used to come here each summer when he was a little boy, and we retrace their steps – to the café where they used to have breakfast, to the secluded beach at the end of a winding single-track lane where they used to swim. We arrive at the beach in early evening, the sky white with that nostalgic light you get in between seasons, a hint of mellow summer tinged with the crisper drama of autumn. On the sand we disperse: Alexander takes his shoes off and begins to walk towards the other side of the cove, his father settles into a folding chair to read, his mother combs the shoreline for shells. The sea is warm and calm and I strip down to my navy blue suit and get in the water, take a few strokes towards the horizon and turn to look back at the figures on the beach.

The rented cottage is unnecessarily large, three sprawling bedrooms spread across three storeys, so Alexander's godparents drive over from Dorset to stay for a few nights, and we all sit around drinking too much wine in the evenings and too much coffee in the mornings. We've recently decided once and for all to get married in June, set a date, booked a venue, made an appointment at the registry office to give our notice of marriage: it's official now. Everyone is excited for us, our parents, our friends; I sense in them, but also in ourselves, a kind of relief, that now we can actually start to plan, to look forward to what has been until now something too theoretical to have much meaning. The night Alexander's godparents arrive at the cottage they raise a glass to us at dinner, and I am struck by their genuine happiness: I had thought for so long of the decision to get married as something that concerned *only* us, and I had forgotten that our lives are linked to the people *around* us.

All that week I browse wedding dresses online, row after row of long white gowns that I can't afford, am not really tall enough to wear anyhow. In a notebook we make lists, try to calculate how much wine our friends will drink, how much time each phase of the day will take. The wedding takes shape.

The weather in Dartmouth is unseasonably warm. I worry about my half-marathon training, go for hilly runs, do sit-ups and push-ups on the soft carpet of our bedroom. We take a boat to Agatha Christie's house, sit on a grassy hill overlooking the trees and the river below. The air is so soft at times that it almost hurts, like a last gasp before the chill of autumn sets in. One afternoon Alexander and I walk along the coast path for a few miles; there's a photo of us from that day, a steep drop down to a cove behind us, the sea bright turquoise. Everything is warmed by golden light and we stand close, sunglasses covering our eyes. In the photo I can see the muscles in my arms, subtle as they are.

It's both a beginning and an end, and we're none the wiser.

★

Two weeks later I take a pregnancy test an hour before I'm scheduled to do a session at the track, my last before the half-marathon. Two clear blue lines: pregnant. I check and recheck the information leaflet that came with the test to confirm my own reading of these lines, though it couldn't be less ambiguous. After all this time, somehow it comes as a genuine surprise; it's not so much that I had managed to stop thinking about it, stop wanting it, but that I had begun to get so used to the state of *not-this-month-maybe-next-month* that an actual pregnancy had started to seem like something perpetually out of reach. It was only this morning that all the individual symptoms I had been overlooking arranged themselves into a cohesive narrative. My period was late, I had been feeling unduly heavy and tired lately, especially when running, my breasts were tender to the touch . . . *Oh!* I thought, like a woman in a film, a heavy-handed realisation, and on my way home from a meeting I bought a two-pack of tests from Boots. I will come to hate the neatness of this moment later, the twee-ness of it, but never mind: it's how it happened.

When I see the result I decide that the track can wait, indefinitely. But I also have this smug little thought, retrospectively pernicious: that my body is working better than it ever has before. Athletically, reproductively, I think, it is doing exactly what it is *supposed to do*. I go and lie down on the bed. What now? I think. The evening stretches ahead of me; if I don't go to the track I can make dinner early, I can watch a film, I can get some writing done, or read a book before bed. All of these things feel too small to mark the occasion, but what else is there? I lie there for quite some time, alone and full with the knowledge, feeling it settle in my body, considering what it means not in the grand scheme of things but in banal terms – what foods will I have to avoid now, I guess I'll have to modify my exercise routine, how will I decline a beer at the pub with friends without raising suspicion?

Alexander is at a book launch in London. He texts me at midnight from Soho: everyone is very drunk; somewhere between one bar and another the author has mysteriously disappeared. *Just finishing drinks – heading home soon!* He promises, though I know that 'soon' might mean anything. Mine doesn't feel like news I can text back. Instead I say *Remember we have that doctor's appointment at 9 a.m.!* Still, he doesn't get home until the early hours of the morning, light seeping out from the edges of the horizon, and I don't get a chance to tell him until half an hour before the taxi arrives. I bring him a cup of coffee while he gets dressed and sit on the edge of the bed, trying to hurry him along so we won't be late, but eager not to rush the moment, either. What do you say? I feel self-conscious somehow, shy, as if we're strangers again, not people who live together, sleep together, are about to get married. I stumble my way through a sentence, then show him the stick on which I peed last night, the proof, the record, which speaks for me. He's hungover, maybe still a little drunk, amazed. In the taxi he can't stop laughing, and neither can I. Radio 1 plays through tinny speakers, hits I don't recognise, don't know the words to. I wonder if the taxi driver thinks we're mad; perhaps we are.

The appointment is with our GP, so that he can refer us to the fertility clinic for further investigations. Instead of discussing the referral, we tell the GP that I'm pregnant. He talks to us briefly about what to do next, about what he describes as the small risk of miscarriage, about how to book an appointment with the midwife in a few weeks. He calculates my due date: a week before our wedding date; we'll have to change it, or cancel it, but never mind. He tells us – from experience, not as a doctor, I think – that everything will change, but not in that way that sometimes people say it to make it seem like having a child is a complete surrender of your existing self, or the only truly meaningful thing in life; he says it in a way that makes it seem like an exciting but ordinary possibility, like our life will still be *ours*, just a little altered. As he speaks I think: *we're that couple*. The couple he'll tell another struggling couple about – they'd been trying for a year and a half, I was just about to send them to the fertility clinic, when . . .

As we stand up to leave he smiles and says, 'Welcome to the rest of your life!'

On the street outside the doctor's office we stand in a slant of early autumn sunshine, at a bit of a loose end. We have to get back to work. We have to call the wedding venue, the registry office. We have to tell our parents, who are helping us pay for the wedding and deserve, we think, to know why, just when we were finally starting to move definitively ahead with our plans, we have so drastically altered them. We have to think about the future we want without assuming it's a given, sketch the contours of it, details to be filled in later. *Welcome to the rest of your life!* But really there's nothing to do but wait, nothing to do but keep living exactly as if both nothing and everything is different.

The next day, a Saturday, the weather is soft and warm and we go for a walk at dusk, the light like gold dust on the dried grass, the trees humming in a breeze with the same sort of nervous energy that propels us at some pace round the perimeter of the park. I have a sense of wanting to freeze the moment, the feeling: everything is all right, everything is as it should be, our future is growing inside me. It's the taste of near-perfect happiness, a whisper on the tongue, sweeter for being delayed, and for now at least our innocence protects us from the bitterness of doubt, of fear. A beginning and an end, *the rest of your life*: truly there is no way we will ever be the same as we were before now, no matter what happens, but I am thinking only in this moment of the future, the promise, the child we will hold. On the way home we stop at a pub and sit in a corner by the window. At the table to our right is a couple cradling a newborn baby, their first real outing, they are telling their friends, since the birth, and at the table to our left another couple, the woman visibly pregnant, are making preparations, listing items they haven't bought yet – *cot, car seat* – and laughing nervously, and though they can't see it yet we belong here, in just this corner of the pub, with just these people.

3

A Question Mark

The bald conclusiveness of a positive pregnancy test draws a clear line between yes/no, this/that, knowing/not-knowing. For a moment at least it clarifies everything, or distils it, into a single and irrefutable piece of knowledge. This certainty, when it comes to the body, is rare (later a doctor will tell me: *if everything in medicine were as reliable as a pregnancy test, my job would be a lot easier*), so I hold on to that piece of knowledge, which is proof of my own productivity, for as long as I can. But doubt, worry, have a way of threading their way through even the solidest conviction. Threat is everywhere: a light fever, an undercooked egg. Indeed the more I read the more I realise how fragile a pregnancy is, how it isn't as simple as a positive test and a baby nine months later, which is something I suppose I always knew in the abstract but never had any real frame of reference for before. I was aware that some of my friends and acquaintances, for example, had had miscarriages, but I had not until now really understood what it meant, in both practical and emotional terms, to have to hold an awareness of this terrible possibility always alongside a hope, a longing, for it not to happen to *you*. Most of what I know about pregnancy, in fact, comes from fiction, from books, films, TV: the way certain signifiers – wooziness, weakness, nausea – are used to suggest a pregnancy before it is confirmed; the way, once it *is* confirmed, a woman must somehow both alter her behaviour drastically and hardly at all, vomiting copiously into a bin at work seconds before giving a presentation just as if nothing is amiss, but studiously avoiding, suddenly, a whole litany of food and drink; most of all the way a baby is almost always the inevitable result of a pregnancy. The plain fact of it – that at least one in four pregnancies end in miscarriage, perhaps more, since sometimes a woman might miscarry before she even knows she's pregnant – had somehow eluded me, or else I had somehow failed to think of it in tangible terms.[1] What does that statistic actually *mean*, practically speaking? It means that nothing is a given. It means that there are people – a lot of people – for whom the result of a pregnancy is not a baby. It means that even the purest elation is often shaded, especially in the early weeks, when miscarriage is most likely, with fear.

I develop a set of superstitions for protection; certain shirts for luck, certain routes home from the library or the grocery store, certain songs skipped or repeated. An aping at control. And for a while everything is normal, in the sense that nothing is normal, in the sense that I feel slightly ill, weary, a little as if I am *not myself*. My overriding emotion is happiness, but there is also a part of me that feels as if I have become separated somehow from my body, as if it is acting of its own accord, and the thinking part of me is just along for the ride. There are psychological adjustments to make – I have to play the phrase *I'm pregnant* over and over to myself to believe it; I have to think about what is good for me not in terms of my body only, but also in terms of the invisible body-to-be inside me. There are physical symptoms, too, though they are mild (another thing I didn't realise: that while some pregnant women are indeed debilitated by illness or weariness, not everyone is). I am never actually sick, though I am dogged by a whisper of nausea that asserts itself at odd times and leads me to keep a pack of digestives on my bedside table. I can feel a largeness, a tenderness, to my breasts, and although I know it's far too early for the pregnancy itself to show I feel fuller somehow, heavier than I was before I knew, as if the knowledge itself has some weight or substance to it.

This is not an unpleasant feeling – because it is a novelty, and because the pregnancy is so unequivocally desired – but it is hard to escape a sense of uneasiness as I walk familiar routes around the city with my headphones in and feel every encounter between feet and pavement to be different now, because I am differently bodied. What I have is a sense, visceral and unignorable, that my body no longer belongs wholly to me – and in a way it doesn't. As I walk I feel not exactly a 'we', but a blooming plurality, an 'I and . . .', perhaps, the assertion of a possibility taking physical form. Where once I occupied my mind during walks with long, elaborate daydreams, there now seems to be no room for anything other than the immediacy of experience and the planning and execution of the tasks of my own daily life. I take to listening to radio shows and podcasts, tuning out my external surroundings and internal circumstances, focusing on the minute details of, say, a true crime story, losing myself in the voice of the presenter.

Geographers write about the inseparability of the body from our experience of place: we sense places, are bodily present in them, see them, hear them, smell them, move within them. How else do we know a favourite room or city or mountain trail? The body, as Tim Edensor writes, *is the means through which we experience and feel the world.*

To which he adds: *bodies are not only written upon but also write their own feelings upon a space in a process of continual remaking.*

What I am struck by in the delicate earliest weeks of pregnancy is that I am being both made and unmade; rewritten. The pregnancy is largely unspoken of: we have told our doctor, and our parents, which perhaps lends it a weight in the world that it wouldn't yet have had we not told anyone, but day to day I move through the hours without anyone but us knowing, because the pregnancy is still invisible. When I stand in front of the mirror I see nothing different, but nothing the same, either. When I go to the pool the place of it has shifted, though the change is microscopic, under the surface. On a quiet morning I watch the play of sunlight on the bottom of the pool and I am in a foreign country. In the changing room, pulling off my wet suit after a shower, I am self-conscious for the first time – *can they tell?* But I want them to tell, even though there's no way they possibly could, even though when I think of it I have the sense not so much of the world tilting on its axis but of the axis itself having drifted elsewhere. I smile knowingly at a visibly pregnant woman undressing and she looks away, uncomprehending or embarrassed or both. *I* am the foreign country, or else I have lost the map of this place. Walking home, along the same roads I have always taken, the green of the trees fading into yellow, I feel somehow both lonely and plural.

And then.

One morning, a few weeks after our appointment with the GP, I wake up and feel my old self again – that is to say, not ill, not weary, not plural or novel – and that evening I experience some mild pain, a quick gush of blood which soon slows to an ambiguous but ominous trickle, and a sense of doom. I am not sure what the appropriate reaction is: denial? Despair? I cannot summon the energy to cook or even to eat dinner; although it is still early I retire to bed, lying on top of the duvet, curled into a question mark. Alexander lies down next to me, his body settling around mine. He tells me the things I both want and don't want to hear: that it's OK, that we don't know for sure that anything's wrong yet, that he loves me. He's meant to be playing football in twenty minutes. Do you want me to stay? he says. I'll stay with you. No, I say vehemently, as if this is in fact an uncharitable suggestion, you should go, you should play, what can you do at this point, what can I do? Nothing. Even after he's pulled his socks over his shinpads, laced up his boots, he hesitates at the door: are you sure you don't want me to stay? I don't want you to stay, I say emphatically. If I were being honest – with him, with myself – I'd say exactly the opposite: stay, please. Instead I lie back and stare at the wall for an hour until he gets home and we go to sleep.

The next morning I call my GP, who arranges an emergency scan for me at the hospital. The soonest the scan can be done is in two days, so in the interim period I carry on as usual: I go to meetings, answer emails, run errands. It's not as hard to do this as I would have imagined it would be, and after all, what choice do I have? But it's also indicative of the ongoingness that will characterise much of the next two months.

I would have imagined, too, that a miscarriage was a definite thing – yes/no, this/that, knowing/not-knowing – a neatly shaped happening with a beginning, a middle, a definitive end, each closely following the other. Women say, 'I had a miscarriage', and until now I have always heard their experience as being something contained, even while brutally uncontrollable: all those stories of blood-drenched bathroom floors, of unimaginable agony, of horror and shock, of sadness and then resolution (often in the form of a baby arriving a year or two on, as if some consolation must always be offered): what I understand now, of course, is that these stories are told retrospectively, packaged in the way that all stories, to some extent, must be. But when I phone the doctor I'm unsure, grammatically speaking, how to phrase my concern: do I say to him that I have *had* a miscarriage, that I'm *having* one, that I'm worried I *might have* one in the future? The idea of the miscarriage in progress perplexes the part of me that imagined that this is a thing that can only happen privately, violently, suddenly, because it is a thing that is happening without much noise at all, and meanwhile here I am transcribing an interview, here I am meeting with a freelance client, wearing a new skirt I bought yesterday from the charity shop, here I am buying groceries and planning dinner, with nothing but a question mark inside me.

Alexander and I take a taxi to the hospital for the scan; it's early morning and the driver is playing loud Pakistani pop, which is somehow soothing, and drowns out my own thoughts. In the waiting room Alexander scrolls restlessly through his phone. A little plastic radio on a cabinet in the corner of the room is pumping out cheerful tunes punctuated by cheerful radio host banter. I take my book from my handbag and lay it on my knees, open at my marked place. Knausgaard, *A Death in the Family*. In his younger-self narrative, the author's father has just died, while in his current-self narrative, his partner is heavily pregnant, lumbering around, practically bursting with new life. But I cannot read on. I become fixated on a single paragraph, a description of a piece of artwork, which strikes me as incomprehensible. I read it over and over again until my name is called.

The scan reveals an embryo with no heartbeat. I lie on the bed, naked from the waist down, a blue plastic sheet draped over my legs. Alexander holds my hand while the ultrasound technician swirls a wand around inside me, talking us through the image of my uterus on the screen. It is illegible to me – darkness, light, hazy shapes – but to her the meaning is crystal clear. I'm so sorry it's not the news you were hoping for, she says. She gives me a wad of tissue to wipe myself with before leaving the room to let me get dressed. She leads us back to the waiting room, which is fuller now, no one making eye contact, the radio still humming; a doctor will see you soon, she says, to talk to you about what happens next. 'Soon' is an ambiguous word, and time becomes difficult to perceive; we are there for what feels like both an eternity and an instant. I take my book out again, stare again at that same page; Alexander unlocks his phone, moves his finger across the screen in a kind of robotic motion.

Sometimes these things resolve naturally, the doctor says when we are finally called in to see her; sometimes intervention becomes necessary, or desirable. She schedules me for another scan the following week, so we can monitor whether there's been any change: in other words, whether the products of conception, as the embryo is now known, have been partially or even wholly expelled. After the scan, she says, we can decide how to proceed; you don't need to make any decisions now. Good, I think, though I'm a little hazy on exactly what kind of decision I might be called upon to make; she has described the various forms of intervention but I can't quite situate them in relation to my own body, my own *products of conception*.

She is very young, the doctor, soft-spoken, apologetic. She says to call if anything changes before my next appointment, if I have any concerns. She gives me a business card, circles a phone number that's operational 24/7. To minimise the risk of infection, she adds, seemingly as an afterthought, you shouldn't take baths or swim.

No swimming. Of course. But I am thrown by the thought of this: the removal of the most obvious physical coping mechanism I have for dealing with what is essentially an entirely uncontrollable physical situation. I realise I've said this out loud without really meaning to. A silence falls, either respectful or uncomfortable.

I'm a swimmer too, the doctor says suddenly, as I'm standing to leave, abandoning, briefly, her professional distance. I'd hate not to be able to do it.

After the appointment we walk to a Starbucks near the hospital. It's dark and anonymous inside, and smells of sweet pastries and wee. I order a latte, two shots, why not, and we sit at a counter at the window, watching buses trundle by. It's mid-morning and the place is full of new mothers and their prams, though occasionally someone in scrubs or a suit hurries in and then out again. Alexander texts his boss to say he won't be coming in to work today. Not just the day but the month, the year, stretches out before us, suddenly open. What will we do with it? What can we do? The coffee is too hot, tasteless, the milk burned, but I suck it down in a rush, turning the inside of my mouth furry. I remember out loud that we never got round to cancelling the registrar, the wedding venue, that after all we won't need to change the date, we can pick up where we left off. I feel myself begin to rewrite the map again, to slip in and out of familiarity with myself and my surroundings. There's a simplicity to it all, underneath the ambiguity, the anguish, that makes me almost giddy: for what is this but a reversion to my natural state, a return to old routines?

A thought – terrible, comforting – hits me square in the face then, that there's *relief* to be felt. The awful thing, the dreaded thing, has happened, and I need no longer fear it. I hate myself for feeling this but can't let go of it, either, because I think it's a way forward, a way out, a small tremble of light.

The second scan is no more or less enlightening than the first: there is still an embryo, there is still no heartbeat. No change, in other words: an unwanted stillness.

The doctor gives me a leaflet, which outlines in clinical language the three ways of managing a miscarriage when pregnancy tissue remains in the womb: expectant, medical, surgical. The first is the wait-and-see approach, taken on the assumption that the tissue will pass naturally out of the womb with time. The second involves taking a course of medication to stimulate the passing of the tissue out of the womb: a potentially painful, lengthy, and often messy process, not always entirely effective, sometimes necessitating the third approach anyhow, which involves surgical removal of the tissue.

I still don't know how to decide what to do, so I put it off: if nothing's happened in a few weeks I'll opt for some kind of intervention. I want above all to trust my body to do whatever needs doing, but already it's betrayed me once, so what do I know?

Still no swimming, obviously, the doctor says sadly. Otherwise, proceed as normal.

As normal. Nothing is normal, I start to think – but then again, in a kind of terrible way, everything is normal again, isn't it?

4

The Geography Closest In

The present-tenseness of the event, the miscarriage, which is not so much an event as a continual unfolding of uncharted territory, a vast grey area, makes it virtually impossible to talk about in any way that makes sense of what is actually happening. I don't know what to tell people because the language I have is not elastic enough to encompass something which is past, present and future all at once. So I do what the doctor suggests: I proceed more or less as normal, going to meetings, going to the supermarket, scrolling mindlessly through Twitter, doing the laundry, eating, sleeping, working. I let myself lose track of time. At one point, in a notebook, next to a to-do list, I write: *The calendar is a kind of enemy, reminding me of the facts of things, the time it is actively taking to go through this process of miscarriage.* I take to walking – long, slow strolls at the very edge of dusk, through parks and quiet suburban neighbourhoods that smell of woodsmoke and exhaust fumes. I feel my muscles going slack, and an irrational fear grows daily: *what will my body become while I can't swim?*

My fear is really a form of vanity. I know that with each day or week that passes without a swim my body will start to look subtly different. I'll lose, am losing, the public indicators of my fitness – the muscle, the shape of my arms and legs, the things that say to other people that I'm disciplined, that my body is under control. And I don't want them to see what I know: that nothing is under control, that this body is not working properly, that athletically, reproductively, it is not doing at all what it's supposed to do. Words come to me on my walks, as they used to on my swims. Some of them are obvious. *Why is this happening to me?* I think selfishly, inevitably, as I climb the hill to the park on a soft bed of wet leaves, fresh-fallen after a night of howling wind. But other things, too, drifting like the smoke and the fumes. Disobedience. Betrayal. Softening, slackening, slowing. *Undisciplined.* Back at home, in my notebook, I write: *I guess I feel disconnected from a part of myself. Not that I'm not still the same person or can't be again, but that for a while I and some other part of me are not quite coinciding.* I'm talking about the swimming, not the miscarriage, or at least ostensibly I am. I have a deep sense of geographical dissonance, like a dream of a familiar place in which the location of everything is slightly wrong, so that you round the corner and suddenly come upon a street that should be miles away, or discover that all along there has been an extra room in your house.

One Sunday afternoon, sitting in a booth at my local pub, I see a woman I used to see most weekday mornings at the pool; she always wore a bright pink cap, a navy swimsuit. She's about my age, sitting with a friend, eating lunch. Perhaps it's her local too, I think, for the first time realising, stupid as it sounds, that these people I've been brushing up against at the pool are people with lives outside that context, just like me.

Occasionally I log on to Facebook and check the triathlon club page. I look through the list of times from a recent 400-metre time trial, spotting familiar names, noting the improvements, and wonder how much I, too, could have improved by now. For a moment I'm gripped by something which feels a little like jealousy but isn't quite – desire, perhaps, something almost carnal. But then the desire, or whatever it is, fades: I'm here now, and maybe, if I can admit it to myself, I'm actually a little relieved that I'm not sweating away in a pool, that I don't have to worry about how fast or smoothly I can cut through the water, how hungry I'll be later, how tired.

*

The poles of the earth have wandered, the journalist John McPhee once wrote: even that which seems most permanent and solid is, in its own way, shifting. It's true literally – think for example of the tectonic plates, the movement of the continents, which still, on average, drift a few centimetres a year apart, *about the rate at which our fingernails grow*, as the geographer Doreen Massey frames it, a reminder that the body is never in stasis either. In other words the whole world is a continual work in progress; *the present is not some kind of achieved terminus*, Massey writes. To underline this idea, she describes the slow movement of what she calls the 'migrant rocks' that came, over the course of millions of years, to form Skiddaw in the Lake District. Solid and eternal as it seems, she says, the mountain is not timeless. Like she and her sister, staying in a hotel in Keswick, it's just *passing through*. It was once elsewhere. It will be elsewhere again someday.

It's easy to lose your footing here, to feel that nothing is solid, but I've always found something comforting about this idea that place is essentially unfixed. The rigidity of permanence would be too much to bear, surely: who wants to be stuck in the same place forever? Who can know and love anywhere and not see that a point on a map is one thing, a living, breathing place quite another?

It's a concept that scales well – if the world is a work in progress, then so too is a city or a street or a swimming pool. So too is the body, which is, after all, as the poet Adrienne Rich puts it, *the geography closest in*; it's the first place, the place we must make peace with – subject, like all places, to the pressures of time, of external rhythms and events, changing from moment to moment, year to year, getting older, bigger, smaller, more or less capable of performing certain tasks, more or less like it was at the beginning.

Sometimes we're in control of that change, or we think we are. Exercise in particular gives us the illusion of power over our own physical futures. Take your recommended thirty minutes of activity a day and stave off all kinds of bodily evil. Lose a bit of weight, add a bit of muscle, establish a routine, live forever, or longer, anyway. The geographer John Bale wrote of exercise as a literal form of recreation: through time, repeated action, *the body is re-created so that it works better.* It incorporates knowledge, becomes stronger, fitter. *Progress.* Maybe next week, or the week after, I'll be faster than I was last week. All it takes is discipline, resolve, another few thousand metres racked up. Most of all denial: of the body that wants, of the possibility of vulnerability or limitation. I think of the Olympic swimmers I watched so closely, of all their talk of sacrifice. Isn't that why I watched in the first place? To see what happens when we write certain kinds of want out of our body, and one singular, possessive, demanding want *into* it: to be the best, the fastest, the one standing on the highest platform of the podium?

Mostly, though, if we're honest, it's the changes in our bodies that are in control of us, not the other way round. The fact of the matter is that not that long ago, my body was capable of running 13.1 miles, of swimming 3,000 metres without complaint; not that long ago, my body was actually hosting another body, or the beginnings of one.

And now everything is different, and everything will be different again someday, and different again, and different again.

5

Common Ground

The odd thing about this time, during which I feel myself to be unravelling, being unmade, is that I also feel a kind of paralysis. Every so often I look at the leaflet on my bedside table – *Your Miscarriage* – but every option fills me with such a deep dread that I think the only sensible thing to do is nothing. The process is invisible; no one knows, to glance at me, that anything is different, or changed, or wrong. I can wait, I keep thinking. I can stay here for a while longer.

Then, in early November, our boiler breaks and the rats move in: two events that are unrelated but seem like more than a coincidence, somehow. The boiler means taking cold showers for a few days while we wait for it to be fixed, and heating water in the stovetop kettle to do the dishes. It's a cold snap, frost on the ground in the mornings. Darkness falls early, but I like walking at the edge of night, when the city looks a little different, when shadows seem like half-formed thoughts.

The rats start innocently enough, just one, lying behind the fridge, stunned by something. Alexander kills it with a broom and I carry it outside and fling it behind the woodpile at the very back of the garden. Then one afternoon as I'm making lunch something runs across my slippered foot. Just a mouse, I think for half a second, before my brain catches up. Then there is evidence of them everywhere: things chewed, droppings on the countertops, a flash of movement in a dark corner. For better or worse the invasion seems confined to the kitchen and we keep the door tightly shut, and for a while I maintain that we can deal with it on our own – I grew up on a ranch, I say, I know rodents. We set traps and kill a slew of them but still there are more. One day I come home from the shop and put some large fresh tomatoes on the counter. Half an hour later I return to the kitchen and one of the tomatoes is gone. When I open the cupboard under the sink there it is, on a shelf, with a neat bite taken out of it.

This is the breaking point. It's too much, I say that night, practically sobbing. We pay Rentokil £400 to rip out the back of our cupboards and lay down poison and steel wool and, more crucially, to take ownership of the situation: now it's *their* problem, even though in practical terms, of course, it's still actually ours.

Meanwhile time, much as I have tried to ignore it, is passing and nothing has changed. Tick, tock: it's been a week, two weeks, three weeks. I feel ragged. I want a hot shower and a clean kitchen and to move forward. I open the leaflet again and make a decision at last to have the surgical intervention.

I'm scheduled for a D&C: a routine operation, low risk, quick, I'm assured. D stands for dilation, a widening of the cervix; C stands for curettage, a scraping of the walls of the uterus. They knock you out with general anaesthetic and fifteen minutes later you're done.

The weekend before the procedure, we go to dinner at the house of some friends who have just moved to a village a few miles outside the city. They live in a cottage adjacent to the old manor house, with an orchard and a chicken coop and a gravelled driveway. Before it gets dark we go for a walk, down lanes and across fields, wellies slapping against our legs. My scarf is made of a cheap fabric that leaves trails of white fluff on my coat and my dress. I want to speak but the wind is up and my nose is running and something about the deep blue dusk clouds my thoughts as well as my vision. I watch the other two women, my friends, good friends, walking side by side and catch their voices drifting towards me – *colleague, Christmas, cigarette, quit* – and feel remote not so much from them as from myself. What would I tell them anyway? The same old problem: what tense to use, what language, what expression to put on my face? I let the countryside silence settle around me, moving slowly through the mud, wishing I had worn a warmer coat.

Later we sit down to dinner and wine and I realise, staring uncomprehendingly across the table at someone who is speaking to me, that I still think it's possible that somehow everything will resolve itself, without effort, without intervention: that I will wake up tomorrow or the next day and find that I have without pain or mess expelled the products of conception, or that I will show up at the hospital and they will say oh, we're so sorry, we made a mistake – everything is fine. Not a miracle so much as the only thinkable option. I haven't known what to tell people not only because there's no language but because I'm afraid of the messiness, the wildness of it, the *what now, who knows* of it. I drag a spoon through my raspberry fool and concentrate for what seems like the first time in weeks. One of my friends is talking about her job at an estate agency, how unhappy she is, how worthless it has made her feel to stay there all this time when she knows she doesn't enjoy the work, isn't valued, and I'm struck by something like relief: this is a thing to share just like any other. But still I find I can only say it at the end of the night, on the threshold, standing in the cold night air, the two bay trees at the front of the cottage illuminated by the headlights of our taxi. The wrong moment, of course, but when is the right one?

★

On the morning of the operation we arrive at the hospital at the appointed time and are ushered through corridors to a space with a single line of bright plastic chairs along one wall, below a frosted-glass window. In front of the chairs are two wood-laminate coffee tables on which various out-of-date magazines are splayed. It's described as a waiting room, though it's not quite a room, and people keep walking past at some pace, sometimes pushing gurneys or medical equipment. There are three other women in the waiting room, each accompanied by a friend or partner, each with a small bag at her feet containing the things we've been told to bring: a dressing gown, a pair of slippers, loose comfortable clothing for after. I try not to stare, but I'm curious about them, and there's not much else to look at. One of the other women has the same last name as me; we'll have to be extra careful, a nurse half-jokes, asking me again for my date of birth, issuing me with a pair of paper bracelets, one for each wrist, a neatly folded, faded hospital gown, missing one of the ties at the neck, and a brand-new pair of tight white surgical stockings, still in the package.

After a while the doctor who's going to perform the operation calls me into a room to talk me through what's about to happen. She's too young for the job, is my first thought. She wears skinny jeans and ballet flats and looks like someone I might meet socially, a friend of a friend; we'd wind up in the kitchen, nursing warm glasses of Oyster Bay, discovering that we had more in common with each other than with our host; we'd exchange numbers, never text but mean to. She opens a file – my file – and says, 'Oh, we were born in the same year!'

It occurs to me that I'm looking for common ground – a name, an age – with anyone I can find it with; with the doctor, but also, particularly, with the other women in the waiting room. The doctor reminds me of my life *before*, of what it's like to be an ordinary twenty-seven-year-old woman in skinny jeans and ballet flats, going about your business, but when I look around the waiting room I get a sense, perhaps for the first time, that there are others here with me, others in the same place, swimming in the murky sea of almost-motherhood. *We're the same, these women and I.* I hold on to that thought while the other Ward is told it's time to get ready; she disappears and emerges from the toilet a few minutes later wearing her hospital gown and stockings under her dressing gown. She seems quite cheerful, leaning over to her partner, murmuring something to him, laughing at his response, but then I suppose so do I, making jokes with Alexander about how sexy I'll look in my own gown and stockings.

For the most part I have fixed my anxiety on the general anaesthetic. What if I have a bad reaction, what if I don't wake up, what if, what if: still more things I can't control. When at last I meet the anaesthetist I tell her I'm nervous – an understatement, she can tell, my voice is shaking. She walks me through what to expect. 'I really want to ease your concerns,' she says, serious but sympathetic. How do I explain that she can't, that they aren't tangible enough for easing? As they prep me for the procedure, set up an IV, she asks me questions about my work. Work seems immaterial, but I find myself talking about it in some detail, and then I'm asleep, and I dream something I can almost remember later, like a taste, and when I wake up I am momentarily giddy.

'Do you feel any pain?' a nurse asks me.

'No!' I cry, almost ecstatic. 'I feel drunk!'

I'm given a cup of tea and a chicken sandwich and left to recover in a small hot room. I don't know where the other women have gone; I'll never knowingly see them again. I miss them but at the same time I'm glad that we don't have to watch each other emerge from the fog. While Alexander dozes in a padded blue plastic chair at my bedside I read an essay about sumo wrestlers and suicide on my iPad. Words float and then dissipate: *rikishi, basho, seppuku.* The essay has a strange dreamlike quality that loosens my already feeble grasp of time; a minute later, or an hour, or is it two, a nurse comes and asks if I feel like I can stand up. When I have demonstrated that I am able to walk unassisted to the loo and back I'm discharged by another nurse, who hands me some leaflets and leaves me to get dressed.

Outside darkness has fallen and we wait for a taxi in the car park, the city hushed by a chill. Our house is warm and rat-free and we eat takeout on the couch before going to bed. In a few weeks all the leaves will be gone from the trees, the days will be at their very shortest, I'll stop bleeding, the pregnancy hormones will leave my body, and it will be, I guess, almost but not quite as if none of this ever happened.

6

The Wild

So now I wait. The doctors have said that once the bleeding has stopped, I can resume all the activities that have been forbidden this past month: I can take a bath, have sex, go for a swim.

The impulse to swim comes back slowly; in a funny way I have become used to my new routines, my new state. I keep going on my long slow walks, shuffling through the leaves at dusk. While I walk, I often consider this question of *ability*, the framing of the body as essentially (re)productive. I think of all the kinds of things bodies can sometimes – but not always – do: set world records; reproduce; recover from open heart surgery; adapt to dramatic, traumatic changes like a lost limb or a deep wound. I think of the things we cannot control; of illness, which so often seems to strike out of nowhere, like an enemy crouched in the forest, but which actually comes from within; of the struggle to conceive, which feels like a betrayal of biology.

Above all I think of a thing the doctor told me when the miscarriage was confirmed – 'there's nothing you could have done' – and of how there really wasn't, even if it's tempting to try to assign reason, blame, even if it would be easier in a sense if there *was* some cause, some fault. What ritual, what superstition, could have prevented this? The truth is: none, not a one. When an Olympian misses out on a medal by a fraction of a millisecond, a slice of time so small that I can't even understand it, let alone feel its passing, it isn't because they weren't good enough or didn't want it enough or didn't wear their lucky goggles, it's just the way it is. When a body slips out of the confines of a plan, a *should*, it's just what bodies do sometimes. Why is it so hard for me to understand this? It's inviolable, inevitable. Sooner or later something like it happens to all of us – we get sick, or injured, or tired, or simply older. Haruki Murakami calls this *the honour of physical decline*. Writing about long-distance running, he admits that he can no longer improve his time – he has reached, and passed, his physical peak. In his fifties, facing the prospect of another marathon, he writes: *I don't care about the time I run. I can try all I want, but I doubt I'll ever be able to run the way I used to. I'm ready to accept that.* Time, he says, is just doing its job on his body. It's a privilege, really, to live long enough to experience this – and in any case there's no point in fighting it. Time has been working on the body since the beginning. Since before the beginning.

I remember, during this period of recovery, a line from a review by Kathleen Jamie, in which she writes about the idea of 'wildness'. It is not a concept, she says, which applies only to the remote and dramatic landscapes to which we customarily associate it, but also to much smaller-scale, more mundane places – even to the body itself.

To give birth is to be in a wild place, she writes, *so is to struggle with pneumonia. If you can look down a gryke, you can look down a microscope, and marvel at the wildness of the processes of our own bodies, the wildness of disease.*

When I read this I felt a fleeting, keen sense of understanding, sharp and sweet at the same time: the truth of the matter is that whether you swim laps religiously or walk aimlessly or run ultramarathons or avoid exercise altogether, the body is itself a wild thing – *And in the end,* as Jamie writes, *we won't have to go out and find the wild, because the wild will come for us.*

7

Somewhere Strange

How do we start again, then? I don't just mean how do we start to think about conception again, pregnancy, the possibility of further loss, an awareness which will never leave me now, though there is that. I mean how to get back to routine, to normalcy, to solid ground, when the ground is always shifting? How to rebuild what was unmade, when it can never be built in exactly the same way again? A beginning, an end, the rest of your life: there is no way to go back to *before*. We are here now, irretrievably *here*, somewhere new, somewhere strange.

I think I probably won't renew my triathlon club membership in the new year. I've lost track of how to measure myself, how to assess progress, what progress would even look like. All of my metaphors for it so far have been linear, but the prevailing metaphor of the pool, really, is a loop, a there-and-back, always a return to the beginning. When I swim 1,600 metres I've swum a mile, more or less, but in tiny increments, and I've gone nowhere: I get out of the pool exactly where I got in.

Sometimes in the mornings I lie in bed and think, in spite of all I know, that my body is not working properly at all, that it is a faulty machine. This is not what a body, a woman's body, is *supposed to do*, I think.

But maybe there is no *supposed to*: a thought which is both frightening and liberating, and comes not clearly into my consciousness but as a fuzziness, a feeling, that recedes as I try to grab at the edges of it, give it a shape.

I keep saying to myself that everything will be OK when I can swim again, when I can resume my routine at the pool, but this attitude in itself is a form of denial, as if I could somehow be exactly the same as I was before, as if I would want to be. As if the moment I enter the water again will mark the moment that everything else gets easier, too. When really – like all places, because this is just a place, a place in time – it's all a process.

I think about loving swimming the way you love a country, writes Leanne Shapton. When I read this I think about the way I miss California, which is in the way that you will always miss something that shaped you, even if you left it voluntarily. I think, for a flickering moment, of the pool not as a backdrop but a place in its own right. And I think of my grandmother, ninety years old this year. When she was my age she swam five or six times a week; now it's once a week, twice sometimes – and yet, she wrote to me not long ago, *I've made a little progress on my stroke – some days it feels great!*

I hold on to that line as, on a white-cold December morning, I climb on my bike and roll myself poolward for the first time since before the pregnancy, before the miscarriage, before, before, before. All the way there I am on autopilot. Autopilot, too, in the changing room, where there are new faces among the old, and in the shower, where the mould has changed its pattern. I let the hot water run down my back, stretch my underused arms, reach for, but do not quite manage to touch, my toes. I feel conscious of the thin straps of my old suit cutting into my back in new places, of a stiffness in my shoulders, a slight and unfamiliar anxiety. At the edge of the pool I hesitate for a long time, carefully considering which lane to enter: how much speed have I lost, where do I now belong, is that woman swimming along there slower or faster than me? Starting again: I have no sense of the order of things.

But when eventually I can delay no longer, I get in and push off and speed suddenly and briefly seems to matter very little. For a moment submersion in this familiar water is overwhelmingly about immediate sensation. True, I am not as fit, not as efficient as I have been in the past and might – but might not – be in the future, but I still know how to swim.

The first length is strange; I feel briefly dizzy, though not unpleasantly so – I'm reminded of the exciting disorientation that always followed a plunge from the diving board as a child, not knowing which way was up but trusting myself to surface anyhow. For an instant I feel the water in my habituated body, with its muscle memory (even though some muscles have diminished), which needs no introduction to this place – and I also feel it afresh, in my own new, re-created body. It is 25 metres of thrill – and then I reach the wall and flip and it feels like it always feels, more or less, which is to say, sometimes great, and sometimes a great struggle.

When I get out, for just a second, I feel like a wild animal. My skin tingles, my breath comes hard and fast, I am dripping, slick with water and sweat, and there is no map of this moment, or the next.

Three

Under the Surface

2015–2016

I

A Silence

Years ago, when we were first getting to know each other, a friend of mine told me she'd had a miscarriage. It was spring, the smell of blossom heavy and drug-like on the air. It wasn't warm enough but we sat outside anyhow, in the garden of the house she and her boyfriend rented, on chairs dragged out from the kitchen, drinking bottles of dark sweet Belgian beer and smoking cigarettes that she rolled with quick, practised fingers. It had happened that winter. Her boyfriend was a lot older than her, a double-barrelled ex-banker; they wanted a big family, a farmhouse somewhere, cats and chaos. They had been trying for a few months when she got pregnant, and then— It was awful, she said: she ended up in hospital for a few days, with an infection, feverish, alone. The boyfriend, she said matter-of-factly, was not very nice about it all.

She was the first woman who had shared this kind of story with me in any detail. At the time it struck me as sad, and only sad: I couldn't see my way out of the sadness, beyond it, to something more nuanced or useful. Would they try again? She shrugged, the edges of their relationship already fraying, though it would be a while before it would unravel completely. To be honest I didn't really know what it meant, didn't understand the weight or the excruciating depth of it. But I knew it was important, both the fact of it having happened and the fact of it having been told, and it stayed in my consciousness long after the last of the daylight had faded and I had made my way home and eaten my dinner and got on with my own life.

We never spoke about it again, except once, years later, very briefly. I don't know if I'm remembering the story right, if in my innocence or my experience I've conflated a number of stories, put too much stock in that one afternoon. Maybe it was revealed over several afternoons. Maybe some of the clarity, the emotion, that I've imbued it with has been applied retrospectively. But still: whenever I think of that day now I think of how much usually goes unsaid *until*. How silent we are, most of the time, about the things that might mean the most, to us and to others.

I want to tell the truth, or a form of it, but this involves speaking into a silence, which is really a fear. Sometimes it's easier not to. Sometimes I think I would rather not think of it, let alone say a word. Too messy, too mundane, too sad, or not sad enough. But then again I have often had the sense that I am screaming into a crowded room, only to realise that the room is empty, my voice is silent, and it is always at this moment that I feel most afraid. Sometimes I too have thought: I will wait, I will not speak *until*. Until what? Until it becomes a story? But then what happens to everything in between, which is often the bulk of things anyway, the meat of a story, the mess of the everyday?

What I have learned so far is that something like a miscarriage makes noise, but the noise isn't clear. It's like a hum, a throaty something just on the periphery of your hearing. It sounds like your body trying to say something, but what? *Your body must be heard,* wrote the feminist critic Hélène Cixous, and I feel the urgency of this, now more than ever. And yet the inevitable answer to the inevitable question – why did this happen? – is: we don't know. The most common cause of first-trimester miscarriage is a chromosomal abnormality in the embryo that makes it unviable: usually a chance thing, statistically unlikely to recur, certainly not a thing that can be controlled. There's no deeper message there, nothing to interpret. The noise is just noise, and after a while you cease to notice it except in small moments when something draws your attention anew. Time, the sieve, filters out details. I've been paying bills and cooking dinner and boiling water for coffee and writing in my diary and sweeping the stairs and taking my vitamins and, yes, going to the pool, and all the while, *tick, tock,* time has been passing: a week, two weeks, a month, two months, six. Nine.

★

In June, a week after what would have been my due date, Alexander and I get married. I am struck by my own surprise at the experience. For a long time I resist the idea that I want a conventional wedding, or that I will enjoy the process of planning one; I let Alexander take on the brunt of the organisational burden, let him make spreadsheets, calculate costs and quantities, focus my energy on more frivolous things: what I'll wear, what colour lipstick, heels or flats. But it is hard not to be swept up by his enthusiasm, and in fact the wedding itself is *fun*. Well, of course it is: really it's just a big party with lots of people we love. My dress is 1930s lace; a florist friend makes my bouquet, sweet and heavy to hold; in the midst of the ceremony I'm in such a hurry to agree to the marriage that I step on the registrar's lines, which sets everyone laughing. A friend reads a poem by Naomi Shihab Nye: *happiness floats / It doesn't need you to hold it down.* It's a warm grey day and it starts to rain just after the ceremony. At the reception I drink a little too much Crémant du Jura, at dinner a little too much Grenache; later Alexander and I dance until we sweat, and I share a cigarette with a friend after my parents have gone back to their hotel.

At the end of the night Alexander and I bundle up the remaining guests into taxis, then call one for ourselves. It will be a few minutes, the operator says, so in the meantime we stand in a pool of lamplight in a deserted dead-end alley, waiting, smelling the rain-wetted tarmac, feeling a breeze wafting off the river, and it is a moment like the first good, relaxed breath you take after a hard swim or a fast run, where physical pleasure meets a kind of psychological relief, where possibility is implicit, felt rather than thought, and everything coheres simply into a *now* that has no beginning and any number of potential endings.

2

Switchbacks

Later that summer, we fly out to California for our honeymoon. We spend a week on the ranch, about a mile down the dirt road from my parents; their neighbour, an architect, has offered us the use of his house, which is small but perfectly formed, everything delightful, deliberate; polished concrete floors, a tomato-red fridge, an outdoor shower with a shelf on which to place a cup of tea in the morning or a bottle of beer in the evening. From the low bed we look out through the window each morning at the line of oaks and sycamores marking the route of the summer-dry creek bed that snakes down the canyon towards the sea. The landscape is familiar to me, it is home, and yet there is something different about it, too: because I have been away for so long, because, perhaps, I am seeing it with fresh eyes, because here we are, a married couple, on our honeymoon. It's not that marriage has fundamentally changed me, or him, or how we are together, exactly, but I'd be lying if I said I didn't feel somehow altered nevertheless, and it is exciting to retrace my childhood steps down the canyon, to swim at the same beaches I swam at as a teenager, to sink my feet into the hot sand, smell the dry grass and the cowpats, feel the cooling kick of a breeze in the evenings.

From Santa Barbara, we rent a car and drive south and east, across the desert. We spend a night in Las Vegas; neither of us has ever been and we are curious. We arrive at the Bellagio at nearly 9 p.m., and there's a long queue for the check-in desk.

93

When we get to the desk we tell the receptionist that we have just got married, we are on our honeymoon, and he looks at us so wearily and so utterly without interest that we get the message immediately: we will get no special treatment. Who here *hasn't* just got married? Who here *isn't* on their honeymoon? And anyway if they aren't already they soon will be: the brides-to-be with their white sashes and flashing tiaras, the grooms-to-be in custom-made T-shirts, the lurid lure of the late-night wedding chapels with their package deals. The receptionist hands us a key card, checks his watch, brightens a bit. 'If you hurry,' he says, 'you might just catch the buffet before it closes!'

From our room, the biggest hotel room I have ever stayed in, we can see swimming pools below us, the lights of the city, a blackness beyond representing the desert. We walk along the Strip for a while, feeling the press of the crowd. We pass a parade of people with cardboard signs: *please help*; *need money for food*; *need money for weed*. We stop for $1 beers at a dive bar where you can gamble on a screen while you wait for the bartender to pour your PBR into a grubby glass.

Back at the hotel Alexander takes out $100 in cash. He settles at a blackjack table, relying on the relative novelty of his British accent to compensate for the fact that he does not actually know what he's doing. The dealers are stone-faced, in ill-fitting uniforms, and the other players seem to be taking it all very seriously. While Alexander slowly but steadily loses his $100 I stand behind him on the casino floor and allow waitresses in short skirts to bring me free beers. Everything has a mechanical, industrial feel, the slot machines being worked like a production line, the constant procession of tourists like the shuffle of shift-workers at the end of the day. I don't know what time it is when Alexander's stack of chips finally dwindles to one, which we pocket as a souvenir: the hours have no meaning here, at 8 a.m. it is just the same as at 8 p.m., the ambiguous lighting, the fug of smoke. We go to sleep in the giant bed and wake up early, in spite of having been up late. I watch the dawn shadows recede, revealing the sprawling hotel swimming pool below us, empty at this hour, though the deckchairs start to fill as we dress.

After breakfast we escape the city. We spend the next week driving deeper and deeper into the strange, hot, dry landscapes of the American Southwest. We stay with an old family friend in Utah, a wiry, reclusive gem-carver who loans us his tent and gives us a small envelope of cash as a wedding gift. We stop at diners, convenience stores, Hopperesque gas stations with pumps painted fire-engine red; we hardly speak with anyone, a lazy hello maybe, a thanks-have-a-nice-day. We visit assorted canyons – Zion, Bryce, the Grand – at each one thinking how many canyons can you possibly look at, and then finding our breath caught in yet another long, slow *wowwwww*. I'm continually amazed by my own inarticulacy, my inability to put anything other than a sound to these places. *Wowwwww* at the sheer drop down into green valley from Angel's Landing, *wowwwww* at the sun setting over Point Imperial, *wowwwww* at the terracotta-army hoodoos pointing at the sky. *Language is always late for its subject*, writes Robert Macfarlane, but my language seems to have been lost somewhere along the way, or got lodged deep inside.

If I'm honest, totally honest, I am not thinking about how to describe what we're seeing, or feeling. I'm not thinking about tomorrow or yesterday, about the due date that was just before our wedding date. I am not thinking about my impending PhD deadline. I am not thinking about the question mark, the unknown outcome of our decision and desire to have a baby. I am not even thinking about the swimming pool, not missing it, because it isn't here. It is almost like I have slid back into my 'old' life, before I was weighed down by *almost* and *maybe* – except that this is not quite true; it is not really like this. I am merely in a state of suspension. I feel as if I am skating along the surface of things, as if there is no before, no decision, no after. The landscape does this to me, flattens my mind, erases the impulse to dig deeper. Sometimes we are just driving down the same straight highway for hours with no one else in sight, cruise control set at 70 miles per hour, the air conditioning on, the music loud, saying little except to remark on the emptiness of the roads, or to wonder where the next gas station is, where we might grab a snack.

We punctuate the driving with hikes, mostly hikes with hills, hikes that make you work for the reward, so that you feel the landscape not just in your legs but also in your lungs. Switch-backs become a kind of ritual – like a pilgrimage, Alexander says, as we back-and-forth our way towards Angel's Landing. Like swimming laps, I say. Like any repetitive, meditative action: a kind of communion with place. I think about this as I walk: what does my body know – climbing this hill, treading this path? My trail running shoes, purchased almost a decade ago, soles worn thin, give me close contact with rock and soil, and I prefer them to my hiking boots, even if I'm less protected, ankles occasionally twisting, giving out: somehow not a sign of precarity but an underline, an emphasis – *this* is the terrain, the topography. You feel it most keenly when you misjudge it, when the surface interferes with your inertia.

Before we left I'd become interested in the phenomenological idea that the body has some knowledge all its own: muscle memory, movement ingrained through repetition, a reaching out into the world, pulling it into us. A knowledge *in our hands*, Maurice Merleau-Ponty wrote: the knowledge that comes from a lifetime of climbing the same hill each afternoon, or moving through the rooms of a beloved house, or of swimming up and down a lane every morning, a knowledge born of familiarity with actions, with surroundings. Linguistically this is tricky territory, because it relies on the individual, on the senses, on things which we are not good at describing even in casual con-versation. What does it feel like to climb a mountain? To wade into a lake? To brush against your husband's arm accidentally while you stand at the bar, and then to pause there, very close, so that you can smell the sweat on each other? To put a cold bottle to your lips on a hot afternoon, to let the moisture linger on your fingertips?

It's why it's so difficult to tell a doctor that we think something's wrong when there are no specific symptoms to point at except a lack, a fear: we have no shared vocabulary, really, for what it is to be in our own skin.

A family friend, a photographer, had open heart surgery when he was a young man. Before the operation he set up a camera and asked the doctors to take pictures while he lay there, inert and open. I have never seen the images that resulted, but I have always been fascinated by this story, because while I can't say for certain what impulse led him to have the photos taken, I can understand that the temptation to see inside yourself like that, simply and literally, would be very great indeed. The truth is we know very little about the workings of our own bodies, and what we do know is mostly clinical, factual, based on someone else's anatomy, based on guesswork, guidelines from a textbook, statistics, likelihoods, or else on our own family history, as if our past will write our future. Often, by default, what we think we know about bodies in general is based specifically on *men's* bodies, with potentially deadly results – one study found that women in Britain are 50 per cent more likely than men to be misdiagnosed after a heart attack, partly because so many of the relevant medical trials featured primarily male participants.[2] For all the marvels of modern medical science, the tools and tests, the X-rays and MRIs, the body is still a fundamentally mysterious domain, especially on an individual level. All the invisible processes, the ripplings and rumblings beneath the skin: if we're lucky, we'll never see any of that internal stuff. Most of us will never know what our own hearts look like, and even if we did, what would we do with that knowledge, except to carry it like a weight?

I've been thinking about a question Robert Macfarlane asks in one of his books, about *how to represent perception in language,* when perception and place are so intimately linked, when our bodies are the main instrument with which we both experience and express place. When I think about the swimming pool in particular I come up against this difficulty: that the primary way of interacting with it is through the medium of the body, through touch and taste and sound, through the way the water feels on the skin, the way the skin feels in the water. It is hard to articulate what exactly this is, what it means, in words that other people will be able to relate to.

The French poet and philosopher Paul Valéry wrote of swimming that *I take the water in my arms, I love it, I possess it, I give birth with it to a thousand strange ideas.* Through the water, he went on, *my body becomes the ready instrument for my mind,* and if I think of it like that it seems to me that the urge to swim is a creative, a generative urge. I think of the way ideas sometimes clarify after a swim, or coalesce; the way the repetition seems to engender some kind of building-up – of muscle, of experience or understanding. I recall Hockney's interest in the challenge of representing water: *a formal problem,* is how he put it. My impulse has always been to try to write my way analytically through these questions of form and representation, an academic impulse. But if I think about the way *water can be anything,* the way almost, maybe, can be anything, I wonder if this is the right approach, if there's some other language I should be trying to use, or better yet, some other source I should be listening to.

The night before the wedding I had lain in a hotel bed, a little buzzed on the bottle of cheap champagne my best friend and I had drunk earlier, reading Nan Shepherd's book about the Cairngorms, *The Living Mountain.* Just before I drifted off I folded over a page with a sentence that had caught my eye: *Water is speaking.*

It reminded me of something the Olympic swimmer Ian Thorpe describes in the opening to his autobiography. Writing of what it feels like for him to dive into a pool, how he settles into a rhythm no matter how fast or slow he is going, he indicates a process of feeling his way through the water, and feeling the water's way around him: *I try to work out how the water wants to hold me*, he writes. *I listen for any erratic movement which means I'm not relating to the water and I have to modify my stroke.* The body as instrument, the body as author. The body corresponding with and through the water. *I don't need someone to tell me that my stroke looks great or that it looks terrible*, Thorpe says, *because I have an inner sense of the water and the environment is already communicating with me.*

Shepherd's relationship with the landscape she writes about, which I have begun to think of as *hers*, is physical, visceral. She listens and watches, touches, smells, walks barefoot through the heather, lies down close to the earth, *under me the central core of fire from which was thrust this grumbling grinding mass of plutonic rock.* The mountain is at times indistinguishable from her body, or rather her body seems to *become* the mountain. *Slowly I have found my way in*, she writes. Then she adds: *If I had other senses, there are other things I should know.*

Perhaps, I think, rather than worrying so much about what the body, my body, can *do*, focusing on how it performs in its various functions (as swimmer, as woman), I ought to think a little more about what it feels, what it knows.

I want to tune in, I decide. I want to listen.

After the canyons we make our way back west, into California again, Yosemite, the Sierras. On the penultimate day of our trip we find ourselves in Lone Pine, near Mount Whitney, the highest peak in the continental United States. We have a beer at a bar on the main strip, where we find ourselves sitting shoulder to shoulder with another couple who are also on their honeymoon. They got married on the same day we did, it turns out, a strange coincidence. Later we set up our tent in the hot dusky evening light at a campsite a few miles out of town. I have been here before; I am chasing a shadow of myself, as a child, camping with my parents, hearing the tinkle of the creek that runs through the site, and later as a teenager, on a school trip, sleeping out under the stars, giggling late into the night about who we fancied. Now we grill thick steaks over the fire and eat them in darkness, headlamps flickering over our plates, then climb into our sleeping bags and lie listening to the wind dusting the tent, alert to our fears – every shadow, every sound, a potential bear, or some other unnamed enemy – but too tired to take them seriously.

In the morning I wake early to pee. I get the stove going and wait for the water for coffee to boil. The wind pushes itself against me, blows the beetles from my hair, but the day, barely even light, is already hot, and there's a quiet that's almost eerie, as if we're the only campers here, which we may as well be. Later we'll hike up to Lone Pine Lake, elevation 10,000 feet, which is as far up the Mount Whitney Trail as you can go without a permit. The air will be different there, the lake a mirror. There will be a couple of other people around, other hikers, wading into the water until it brushes their knees, but no one will be speaking much. While Alexander wanders along the edge of the lake I will sit and eat an apple with my legs dangling off a rock, looking into the blue.

The most vital thing that can be listened to here is silence, Nan Shepherd wrote of the mountain, and perhaps this is true of all places.

3

Drought

We are, at this point, not actively *trying* for a baby, but we are not *not* trying, either: another liminal space. I have not gone back on the pill. For a few months leading up to the wedding we used condoms, to eliminate the additional stress of ambiguity, of possibility, but there's no need for them now, not out here in the post-wedding world. We can re-enter the realm of almost, of maybe, though perhaps I am reluctant to do so, perhaps it has been more of a respite than I thought not to have to wonder each month whether everything or nothing is about to change. So no: we are not using protection, but I am also not obsessively tracking my cycles, not trying to predict when I might be ovulating, not thinking of sex had outside that narrow window as a waste. At moments it is even possible to feel as if we are starting from scratch, as if we can disregard the past two years: we are just another pair of newlyweds, enjoying each other's company, enjoying our freedom before embarking on the journey to parenthood. Who knows, perhaps we'll get lucky this time, perhaps it will be easy, why not.

But here's the problem with this place, this repetitive, switchbacked landscape of almost, of maybe: it's a trap, a cage, a sentence that leads you up the mountain but not back down again. Once you arrive here you can only pretend for so long that you came voluntarily, that you haven't lost your bearings. You can close your eyes and imagine you aren't here, and it might almost feel true, for a moment. But eventually you have to face up to the fact: you *are* here. You have been for some time. You may be for longer still. The path out, if there is a path out, is still uncut.

In California, there are signs everywhere of the ongoing drought. At this time of year, late summer, the hills are always bleached, but now there is something different about them. In the evenings, as the sun lowers itself wearily, they begin to glow, not warmly but as if currents of electricity are running up their backs, standing hair on end. The ground is grey, the cars are wheezy and dusty, the wind, when it kicks up, sets everyone's teeth on edge. We are back on the ranch after our road trip, staying with my parents, and on all our minds, I can feel it, is the worry of fire: all it takes is an errant spark somewhere and all this will go up in flames, the house my parents built, the hillside paths I spent my childhood learning and relearning, the sycamore trees I planted and watered and watched for years, until they were far taller than me, the macadamia orchard, the water tanks and wind breaks, all the marks of our presence here.

One afternoon, a few days before we fly back to England, Alexander and I are at the beach, sitting on a picnic bench, watching small waves roll over on the shore, when a deep belly noise rumbles, like a rocket being launched. Then, sun still blazing, droplets hit my feet, my legs. For a moment I wonder what's dripping on me, until I realise that under the ceiling of the sky rain is falling. The storm, such as it is – pushed up from Baja, apparently, all blustery clouds and no real substance – rolls away moments later, over the hills, in a hurry to get somewhere else. Almost by the time I've realised what it is, there's no trace of it.

This ghost rain is not enough, of course. The drought will go on. Farmers will worry about their crops, everyone will worry about fire, in the newspapers they will continue to print strange stories of wild animals coming down from the hills, skulking around houses, hungry, desperate for water. The word *barren* will be planted in my mind. What can grow here? Barren: the word a wasteland. A desert. Dried up.

4

Swimming Sense

Back home in Oxford, we return to work, to old habits and routines. It is August, the city teeming with tourists, the weather unpredictable, hot then cool, rain then sun. I go to the pool the day after we return, jet-lagged, woozy from lack of sleep, eager for the water to wake me up, and after three weeks away there it is, just as it always has been, unchanged, waiting. It's not the open expanse of the Pacific, but still: it's water, cool and soothing after the heat and the dust of our trip, an old friend.

At the pool, most of the women in the changing room are older than me. Because I work from home, I have the luxury of waiting until the pre-work rush hour is over, getting in just as everyone who has an office to get to, a 9 a.m. conference call, a tea round, a barrage of emails, is getting out. The women I swim with are also self-employed, or semi-retired, or fully retired. Their lives are soft and flexible, or seem that way to me. They have started to smile hello to me, a fellow regular. As I get dressed after my shower I listen to their conversations. Often, I notice, they are talking about their children or grandchildren, sometimes with a kind of weary resignation: they are being called upon by sons and daughters to look after babies, to be available and responsible, at a time in their lives when they thought they were done looking after babies, done being available and responsible, at least in that particular way. There's pleasure in it, too, of course, and I see that these moments in the conversation are a kind of communion of fellows.

I am the odd one out, I think. I'm the age of their children. I should be foisting a baby on *my* parents for a weekend, inviting *my* in-laws on holiday with us so they can give us some relief. I wonder what they think when they look at me, these older women, what they think when they smile hello. Can they see that I do not belong? But I have started to feel as if I do, and I find the drift of their voices across the room soothing.

A few weeks after the honeymoon, though, I take a part-time job in an office, to give myself structure, and a stable income, while I attack my PhD thesis once and for all, try to get it done and dusted in the next year. I have to be in the office at nine each morning; I become one of those rushed young women, frantically drying their hair, doing their make-up in front of a steamy mirror. Sometimes I get a glimpse of someone I recognise arriving as I'm leaving, and I feel as if I've been pushed out of time, out of my own life somehow, onto a different track; I see the ghost of myself in the changing room, realise too late how much I have come to depend not only on the water itself but on something more solid – the staidness of routine, the flesh-and-bones women that I almost-know, the feeling of what? Of having a place.

*

Still: I said I wanted to tune in, so I will. Instead of worrying about how fast I am, how far I have time to swim, I think in the mornings about what it feels like to slide below the surface of the water. I think about the cold of it, the wet of it. I think about how sometimes, a few hours after my swim, I'll rest my chin in my hands or rub my palms across my face if I am feeling unsure about how to begin a task, and I will catch a trace of something. Chlorine, but marked by time, diluted by the smell of the hand soap in the bathroom, the shampoo I used in my hair after my swim, the garlic I sliced at lunchtime.

It reminds me, first and most viscerally, of the pleasure of a swim, what it feels like to be in water, the comfort of the environment; if I happen to be somewhere strange or uncomfortable (a dentist's waiting room, a cramped bus) the smell is soothing, a reminder of a familiar place, a familiar state. At the same time it reminds me of my childhood, and not only of the happy carefree hours spent lolling around in cold turquoise pools on hot bright summer days. It reminds me particularly of swimming lessons with an instructor called Char, of whom I was afraid. She had a booming, husky voice that conveyed disappointment or disapproval no matter what it was saying. She always wore a clear plastic visor and had rough, saggy brown skin from too many years of sunbathing, too many years of pacing the deck, barking at frightened children, compelling them into the water, willing them to adopt better, more fluid form. My mother likes to tell a story about how one day I finally admitted to her that I didn't like the lessons: 'Char gives me the same feeling as the sound of my alarm clock in the morning,' I allegedly said. And so I will be in the dentist's waiting room, or sitting on the bus, but also elsewhere, in the past, a big Orange County pool, the smell on my hands reminding me of those lessons during which I grew aware of myself, during which I became afraid, not specifically of drowning, not specifically of the deep end, but of my own bodily limitations. I swallowed water, came up spluttering, clung to the side of the pool and yearned to be back on land. In the car, on the way home, I would be heavy and hungry and sleepy.

Smell is famously evocative; a whiff of anything may, to borrow the phrasing of Yi-Fu Tuan, *call to mind an entire complex of sensations*, in particular those associated with the past. Tuan posits that this may be because *the cortex with its vast memory store evolved from the part of the brain originally concerned with smell* – or because, more simply, our noses as children were more sensitive and *closer to the earth*. It's true, I was closer to the earth once, when I dragged my feet on the hot concrete, reluctant to get in the pool. *An entire complex of sensations*: sunburn, the sting of chlorine in my eyes, the feel of it at the back of my throat, a sense of disappointment, of relief.

You could get lost in sensation. Perhaps that's the attraction, the point: *The great object of life is Sensation — to feel that we exist*, Lord Byron once wrote in a letter to his future wife, Annabella Milbanke. Perhaps especially for Byron, who despite his famed athleticism in water was hobbled by a deformed foot, swimming was a means to sensation (a plinth in Italy remembers him as the 'noted English Swimmer and Poet', placing his prowess in water, rather than on the page, in the prime position). But the work of other Romantic poets, too, often seems suffused with water. Percy Bysshe Shelley, of course, never learned to swim and drowned in a storm off the coast of Italy, but he was drawn irresistibly to water, his *fatal element*, as his cousin Thomas Medwin puts it. (His first wife, Harriet, drowned too, in the Serpentine, *far advanced in pregnancy*, according to a report in *The Times*, two years after they were estranged.) Indeed, the word 'swim', Charles Sprawson points out, recurs in lines of verse from the period: Keats feeling *like some watcher of the skies / When a new planet swims into his ken*, for example, or Coleridge *silent with swimming sense*. Something about the word lends itself to whatever it describes; it has a natural sensuality, a kind of wateriness that allows it to slide in and out of all kinds of meanings, expanding, contracting, adapting, its definition never quite precisely identifiable.

At one point, pursuing a train of thought down an internet rabbit hole, I encounter an entry on Wikipedia that claims that the word 'swim' comes from, among other sources, the Proto-Germanic *swimmanq*: 'to swoon, lose consciousness, swim'. I can find no other evidence that this is true, but it continues to stick with me, because it seems to have emotional if not historical veracity. To swim, to swoon, to lose consciousness: not necessarily in the sense of blacking out, but in some other, more fluid way. To lose consciousness of one way of being, of time and the body as felt on land, but then to (re)gain a new, or different, consciousness: of the body as felt in water; the body's history in water; the expansion and slippage of time. The unknown known, just at the outside edge of perception or understanding.

Silent with swimming sense, I think, slipping in, under the surface. And then a fragment that rolls into my mind and over and over again as if my stroke were generating it: *we exist. We exist.* That's something.

5

Here Be Dragons

Time is still on our side. I am still young. There is no reason to worry. *At least now you know you can get pregnant!* A thing that many people say, trying to be helpful, along with *you're still so young!* It's true, I have to acknowledge. At least now I know. At least I am still *so young.*

Time is still on our side, but it is also still, of course, passing. Autumn now, another autumn, dark and damp, though sometimes there are mornings where the air is so crisp it seems to cut through everything else – doubt, uncertainty, fear – and demand a more immediate attention. Often as I cycle to the pool I feel as if I am *drinking* the air, as if it's flushing through me, alive somehow. But a little part of me thinks: we've had our fun, now back to business. Now back to thinking about ovulation, conception, all the things that might be wrong, or go wrong. Because it has been almost a year since I first conceived, and I have not conceived again, we ask to pick up where we left off, to be referred to the fertility clinic, where they can run further tests, talk about options, next steps.

As part of our referral to the clinic, Alexander's sperm is assessed. He is issued with a small plastic pot with a screw-on lid, as well as an envelope in which to place the pot, and a form to fill out. He must capture some of his semen in the plastic pot and then convey it immediately to the clinic – within about twenty minutes, ideally, the instructions say. The clinic is two miles from our house; not a great distance, but we don't have a car, and the buses, which don't stop particularly near the clinic in any case, are unreliable. He decides to take a taxi, sits rigidly in the back seat holding the pot in its little envelope, with an intense awareness, he says, of the absurdity of the situation.

This story, when we finally start telling it, turns out to be far from unique. We know at least two other men who have also had to carry pots of their own semen to the same clinic in a taxi. Another friend of ours, who lives in a different town and does not have a car, tells us that, not knowing how else to negotiate the specific timings, he produced his specimen in the toilet of a local café and then ran, literally ran, the mile and a half up the road to the clinic.

The crucial role of men in all this is often underplayed. The focus – and the blame – is first and foremost on the woman's body, since this is where the failure of conception seems most evident: a flat belly when it should be round, an empty uterus when it should be full, small flaccid breasts that should be tender and pumped up. Whereas you cannot read a man's body in the same way; the work of his sperm is largely invisible. Indeed the dominant understanding of infertility places an emphasis on the woman to such an extent that we often forget that she is not solely responsible for the outcome of any attempt at conception. I know stories, and you probably do too, of women who struggled for years to conceive before it was finally revealed that the problem lay not with her but with her partner. (And isn't it telling that my first instinct, even now, is to phrase it like this: that it was *she* who struggled to conceive, not him, not them?) Even for those of us who know very well that it takes two, and that it is not always or only women's bodies that betray a hopeful couple, it often comes as a surprise to be reminded that it is not women exclusively who must be questioned and tested.

It's no easier for men, of course, than it is for women to contemplate the implications of infertility: virility is so entwined with narratives of masculinity, just as the ability to bear children is often taken as being *the* defining feature of what it is to be a woman, that it can be difficult to pick apart a sense of self-worth from a reproductive performance over which you have, ultimately, very little control.

It should not, from a practical perspective, make any difference with whom the fault lies: him, me, both of us, neither of us, the result, or the lack of result, is just the same. Perhaps the problem is in thinking through it with this kind of language at all – *fault, blame*, as if there is human agency at work, as if there is a moral failing somewhere. In any case Alexander's test results show that both his sperm count and motility are perfectly healthy. We are relieved, it is one less thing to worry about, another box ticked on the clinic form. But privately I try to imagine what it would be like if the result had been different, if, after all this time, some clarity had come to us not as a result of my body but of his. Would I be resentful? Would it change our relationship, our plan, our outlook?

I think about this because, of course, I am worried that this is how he has come to think of me: as a body only, as a problem to be solved. If we cannot wring the answers from my blood, I think, if the silence of my body persists, will he want eventually to discard me? A conversation I cannot yet have with him: because I am afraid, yes, but also, if I'm honest, because I already know what he will say – that of course he doesn't want, will never want, to discard me, that of course I am more than just a means to an end – and then I will have to face the fact that it is not his judgement of me but my own that's most frightening.

★

The doctor at the clinic, when we finally receive our referral, seems unimpressed by our situation. I can understand why, when he must see so many people who are so much further down a road that we've only just sighted, but on the other hand I want him to appreciate the view from my chair, to give us something like sympathy, an encouraging nod at the end of the appointment. He is keen to list statistics which are in our favour, but in the end acknowledges that perhaps there are enough things stacked against us to warrant intervention. He suggests clomifene, a drug which stimulates ovulation. We agree to try it.

Meanwhile a silence is growing, has grown. I do not tell anyone what we are doing, because it does not seem worth talking about. I pick up the clomifene on an unseasonably warm November afternoon: a year to the day, I realise, since the D&C. I have to have the prescription filled at the hospital, rather than my usual pharmacy, and as I sit in the corridor waiting for my name to be called I wonder, vainly, about how we might announce a much-longed-for pregnancy on Facebook. Would I make reference to the path not being quite as straightforward as we had hoped, as it so often looks? Or would my courage fail me, would I want to put all this squarely behind me, be seen as *normal*?

The truth is this: the language for where we are is hard to pin down. There is no exact way of saying what is wrong with me, or even of determining for certain that something *is* wrong. Everything that has happened so far – which is to say, nothing, and then a miscarriage, and then more nothing – is within the bounds of 'normal', whatever normal may be. On the other hand, statistically speaking, most women my age who had been trying to conceive for as long as we have would be pregnant by now, would have a baby by now, and once again it feels that I'm caught in a place that has no particular name, no particular character or boundary.

Language has become important. It always was, of course, but now I see, or rather feel, the lack of it. I feel where it does not quite meet the edges of what it's describing, and I also feel where my own cowardice precludes me from finding it. The word 'infertility', for example, has always seemed like something definite, certain, foregone, and I have avoided even thinking it, as if I might jinx myself, as if the word might be contagious. But now I see that it is shorthand; it is not certain and solid at all;

it encompasses all possibilities without promising any particular outcome, and if I still cannot use it, I try not to be afraid to see it, to think of it. I try at least to *notice* it, which is a start.

Then, too, there is the rote specificity of medical terminology: words to describe processes and organs I had, until recently, taken for granted, a kind of naming of parts. Luteinising hormone. Thyroid-stimulating hormone. Follicle-stimulating hormone. Progesterone. Basal body temperature. Sperm motility. If I learn enough of these words, will they make a sentence? I start to see the process of undergoing fertility treatment as a kind of mapping, with consultants as cartographers, my body a continent, the labels an attempt at civilising unknown territory – currents, winds, deserts, oceans – and yet there still seems to be an awful lot of *here be dragons* about it.

★

If I were able to, I would try to hold all these thoughts apart from myself for a moment, as if they were nothing to do with me. I would think only of my body as instrument, as author, and I would close my eyes for half a second, coasting down the hill from the hospital with the clomifene in my rucksack, and feel the brush of the wind on my face, the perspiration in my armpits drying, the raggedness of my breath settling, the speed of things. And then I would open my eyes and the afternoon would still be grey, but bright on the edges, and my brakes would squeak as I squeezed them at the bottom of the hill, and when I got home I would lay the pills on the dresser and somehow, somehow, I would imbue them not with too much hope but just enough, and that would be all I would need to feel about any of it.

But we cannot separate ourselves from what we feel, what we hope, what we fear. We cannot retrospectively, or prospectively, tell ourselves how to be.

6

A Double Life

The first month I take the clomifene, it doesn't work. My period arrives a couple of weeks into the new year, unwanted, after all this time somehow unsurprising, in spite of the carefully timed sex we had around Christmas, on the squeaky guest bed at my in-laws' house, giggling, trying and failing to be quiet. Still, it feels as if we're playing a game again: the pills, the ovulation test kits, the scheduled sex. I have a sense of optimism that correlates directly, I think, to how much I feel we are *taking control* of the situation, that is, taking the control away from my body and giving it to the medicine.

The second month, I make a pact with myself that I will only take a pregnancy test if I'm at least two days late. I make this decision at the pool, the morning my period is due. I could have taken the test when I got up, but I chose not to. I chose to come here and act as if nothing is different, because the truth is that in all likelihood nothing *is* different. I get in, I do my 1,600 metres, up and down, up and down. At work I make myself a cup of coffee and allow the trivialities of the day to consume me.

The test, when I take it, is positive. For a moment I am uncomplicatedly thrilled. I am not even surprised: perhaps I had already known, somewhere deep down; perhaps I really have tuned in, learned how to listen. But by the time I have carried the test stick into the bedroom and laid it on top of the dresser another feeling has asserted itself: fear, plain and simple. This time I understand the hugeness of it, the weight of it. No matter what happens, there is no going back; this is the first step on a complex physical and emotional journey. And at the back of my mind, like a fly buzzing in the heat, is the thought: *what if it goes wrong again?* (And what if it doesn't? Either way everything changes.)

Alexander is at work, gets home late; I am half asleep when he climbs into bed and miss the moment to tell him, and the next morning I cycle off to the office before he's awake. There's a part of me, if I'm honest, that doesn't want to share the test result, with him or anyone. I want the knowledge to be only mine for a little while longer: as if, perhaps, by holding it close I can protect us all – Alexander, myself, the tiny speck of possibility that has begun to grow. I float through the day, buoyed by what I and I alone know. I send emails, I go for a walk at lunch, I feel that, although it's still only early February, there might be a touch of spring in the air. I tell Alexander only as we're cooking dinner together that evening, draining the pasta, casually. *I should have said sooner, but I took a test yesterday . . .* But of course he is too happy, or too kind, to care that I kept it from him for a day. Now it is ours, and ours alone, something we can hoard and hold together. The only obligation we have is to notify the fertility clinic; they schedule me for an early scan in a few weeks, so they can check up on the pregnancy before discharging me. Otherwise we have resolved that, unlike last time, we will not share our news with anyone, not our parents, certainly not our friends, until after the twelve-week scan. The silence, I feel, will protect us, though from what I could not say: I already know from experience that loss does not listen to logic, that telling people, not telling people, makes no difference to what happens, or doesn't happen. Intellectually, in fact, I feel that the convention of waiting to announce a pregnancy until the twelve-week mark is problematic: it magnifies the loneliness of early pregnancy, and contributes to a culture that celebrates reproductive success while suppressing a wider awareness of the potential for – the reality of – loss. All the secrecy, the lies, the carefully crafted explanations for changes in behaviour: what good does it do, really, to delay speaking of it? Either way, I think, whether we have a baby nine months later or not, I'll want to tell my friends, my family, eventually. In the meantime all the silence does is underline the strangeness, the uncertainty, of my state, as if I am not really pregnant, not yet anyhow, not until it can be safely announced; the embryo, in essence, exists only in the imagination until it is, statistically speaking at least, safe, though of course nothing can ever be guaranteed, there is no such thing as safe, really.

This is what I believe, at least in theory. And yet now, in the moment, in my fear, I find this intellectual stance challenged, overruled, by my emotional vulnerability. I find myself wanting to use the secrecy as a shield, or is it simply that I don't want to jinx things? That I think somehow, by withholding the information, I can maintain a fragile form of control over an unknown future?

All January I had worked, head down, throughout the cold, damp days: mornings at the office, in a grim 1960s-era building near the train station, and afternoons in the library, puzzling over my thesis. But in February, after the pregnancy test, my tightly wound focus unravels. I take long walks around Oxford on my lunch breaks, listening to music, feeling again, afresh, the strangeness, the newness, of my body, but also telling myself: well, this time it will be different. Entreating myself, more like. Begging. *Let it be different.*

I'm too superstitious to do it myself but Alexander downloads a pregnancy-tracking app on his phone, and each week, at my request, he reads me the update. He finds various items which supposedly correlate with the size of the embryo – a poppy seed, a sesame seed, a lentil – that he lines up along a shelf in the kitchen to mark the progress of the pregnancy. It is hard to imagine, to say the least, what it is that's growing, hard to imagine in what way it can be so potentially complex and yet also the size of a lentil. Hard to imagine, of course, because it's abstract, but also because to imagine is in some way to commit, to affect an attitude of sureness that I do not in fact feel.

Do we dare commit? What would it mean to say *when*, not *if*? What's at stake, since whether I download the app or not, whether I talk speculatively about the future or not, nothing now but time can tell?

When I go for my lunch-hour walks I sometimes catch a reflection of myself in a bookshop window and I think, *it will probably be OK*. This is as much as I can do: not quite a commitment, but almost. An admittance of possibility, at least. A hope, or should I say a plea, a prayer, which is often the same thing. If I cannot say *when*, am still stuck on *if*, if I cannot shake the shiver of involuntary fear I felt when I saw those two lines on the stick, I can do this: I can enact a forced kind of optimism, and hope that eventually, with time, it proves true.

★

Shortly after my twenty-ninth birthday, two days before my scan at the fertility clinic, a few weeks after I take the test, I realise, standing up from the couch to go upstairs to bed, that I am bleeding.

I cannot bring myself to see this as anything but disaster; it seems to follow the form of my first miscarriage so exactly, that first alarming gush of blood, the deep-down conviction that *something is wrong* – even the timing is the same, down to the day. I yell at Alexander, who is saying something from the hallway in a voice that moments ago was appropriate but now feels indecently cheerful, though how is he to know, to shut up. *Shut up*, I say again, and go upstairs, close the bathroom door behind me. Sobered, he follows me up, waits outside. Is it fair, is it right, that I shut him out, shut him up? That my first response is anger – and at who, at what? But a tiny part of me, mean and full of self-loathing, is whispering: *I knew it, I told you so, of course this was bound to happen*, and I am angry at myself, at my body, for the betrayal.

I take the next day off work, claiming illness, though I'm not sure whether this constitutes illness or not, really; I guess there's no reason I couldn't sit at a computer, but instead I lie on the sofa watching films while Alexander, working from home, types abstractedly on his laptop. In one of the films, Rachel McAdams plays an ex-flame of Bradley Cooper's. She's married now, with kids. The film is crap, but watching McAdams in the kitchen with the kids, I am surprised by how much I feel the keenness of a loss. *I wanted that*, I think, already using the past tense, though nothing has been confirmed.

The next day we arrive early for our appointment at the clinic, because what else do we have to do today? All morning I've been imagining the silence, the stillness, of the sonogram. What you want is movement, signifying life. What you get is . . . whatever you get. In the waiting room another couple is seated on the lime-green chairs, and after a few moments a nurse emerges from a room holding a glossy printout, which she hands to the woman. *Oh my goodness, you can really see . . .* the woman says, with something like surprise, even though it is simply a reproduction of an image she'd seen on a screen moments earlier. The couple are giddy. They gather up their things, laughing a little as they button up their coats. They half-smile at us as they step past and I half-smile at them. *Congratulations, assholes*, I think.

I think: *they think we're like them, here for good news. Little do they know.*

But then, in the ultrasound room, the flash of a heartbeat. Movement, signifying life. It's not technically a heartbeat, because the embryo's heart is not yet fully formed, but it's what you want to see at that stage, a flutter where the heart will be. The nurse can see what she calls a subchorionic haematoma, an accumulation of blood between the uterus and the gestational membrane, but the embryo itself looks fine.

It's a good sign, the nurse says to us, to see a heartbeat this early on.

After the scan I get dressed and we emerge, blinking, into the waiting room again. After a few minutes the nurse comes out and gives us our photograph, in the presence of strangers who perhaps are also smiling on the outside and inside thinking *little do they know. Congratulations, assholes.*

We do know! I want to say, to no one in particular. We are giddy, but we are still both, in a way: the couple who arrived full of foreboding, the couple who left with hope and a little photograph folded in an envelope. A double life: that is what this is. I am starting to see that.

★

The nurse has told me that the bleeding should settle in a few days. She used the word *settle* very specifically, and repeatedly, in retrospect I suspect as an alternative to *stop*, because when I get home and start to read online I discover that there are women who bleed for days, for weeks, in early pregnancy, and go on to have healthy babies. Sometimes, in these cases, there's a diagnosis: 'cervical ectropion', for example, when the soft cells from inside the cervical canal are found on the outside surface of the cervix, can cause harmless but alarming bleeding during pregnancy. But usually a reason cannot and will not be identified: it's just *one of those things*, another of the many mysteries of the female reproductive system. It is either nothing, or it is something, and there is no way to know how or if it will resolve except to wait.

If you're worried, the nurse had said before sending us home, or if the bleeding doesn't settle, ring your GP. At the time, in my immense, immediate relief, I had thought: but how cruel would it be for something to go wrong after all this! I discount the possibility on the basis that it's unimaginable. Now in my head I start to compose the forum post I'll write when I'm definitely out of the woods (push the thought away: *but when will that be?*), outlining my experience and the positive outcome for the reassurance of other women to come. *The least I can do*, I think, feeling magnanimous. I have never contributed to these forums, though I have often lurked, reading other people's stories and warnings and assurances; perhaps, I think, I owe these anonymous women something of myself, in thanks, in payment.

As the week wears on the bleeding *settles*, in the sense that it does not get any worse, but it does not go away. I have the photograph, of course, folded in its envelope, as proof. Proof of life. Or of something, anyway. But proof is a drug; how long does it last before you need more? I look at the image, which is more or less meaningless to me, to be honest, except for what I know it signifies, except for what I know I saw, and Alexander saw, on the screen: the flash, the movement, the *everything looks good*. It is not enough, proof, faith, hope on its own. Not for me, anyway, but maybe not for anyone. After a few days I phone my GP surgery and they agree to see me that day. Alexander picks me up from work and we walk to the surgery together. We sit nervously in the waiting room; he holds my hand, which sweats in his. Part of me wants to take it away, to fold in on myself, and part of me can't countenance ever letting go again, even though it's impractical to squeeze through the narrow doorway to the doctor's office hand in hand.

The GP, who is not my normal GP, looks through my notes, speaks to me for some time, feels my abdomen, but this is mostly for show, for reassurance: there's nothing he can determine from here, in his basement office, and he is forthright about this. But he takes my concerns seriously and treats me without condescension or doubt. He calls the hospital and secures me a scan later that afternoon: I know, he says, that sometimes the hardest part of this is all the waiting, the not-knowing.

When we arrive for the scan, the receptionist hands me a plastic receptacle and asks me to fill it with urine. Sitting on the toilet in the dark bathroom, with printed A4 signs peeling from the walls, instructing visitors about where to submit their sample, I have my first grip of real fear. I realise too late that I have been assuming this is for reassurance, assuming the stakes are low, that I am already out of the woods, whatever that means, when all the while things could have been happening inside my body that I've been entirely unaware of.

Watching the doctor looking at the sonogram screen, one hand operating the controls and the other holding the wand inside me, we know immediately that something is wrong, because it takes her some time to speak. Her brow is furrowed and she is silent for so long that it drowns all hope. At the clinic, when we walked in and I said, 'I've been bleeding, I'm pretty sure I know what's coming next,' the nurse practically tripped over herself to speak as soon as she could to give us reassurance: *everything looks good!* This time everything does not look good. A stillness, a silence, again. My hand is slippery in Alexander's; his fingers squeeze mine, or is it the other way around, so hard that it aches. The doctor is kind and I wonder how they keep being so kind, over and over again. As I get dressed behind a screen I can hear her talking to Alexander. She's a senior consultant, as it turns out; this isn't really her job, she's only filling in because of the junior doctors' strike. When I come and sit on the chair next to her computer she tells me she runs the hospital's recurrent miscarriage clinic. To qualify as having recurrent miscarriages, she says, you have to have three in a row. But she'd be happy to see me again, to run a few tests, if I'd like. She schedules me for an MRI, to get a clearer picture of the shape of my uterus, and gives me her assistant's card, so I can ring if I have any questions.

I can't believe our luck, though it's a strange way to think of it. But on the way home what she has said strikes me differently. I think of all her patients. I think, to really start to understand what's going on – to really know, to really speak with my body at any length – I'd have to go through all this *again* – and how could you bear it?

At least I know this: I do not want to wait and see what happens; I do not trust my body; I do not want to waste time. The ungrowing embryo is still there, and I have no reason to believe, based on my symptoms and my previous experience, that this miscarriage will progress differently from the last. I take the rest of the day to consider; Alexander and I are dog-sitting for a friend, and we talk things through as we walk the little terrier, straining at the lead, through the park. But the truth is I do not need to discuss it, and neither does he: now that we know, now that our fear has been confirmed, we can hardly wait to move on, and the next morning, before work, standing outside the office building, I ring the hospital and ask for a D&C. They schedule me as soon as they can, in about a week. They'll scan me again just before the operation, they say, to make sure nothing's changed. In the meantime, no swimming, of course. No sex. No baths. Of course, I say.

After the phone call I go into the office and make a cup of coffee. It is a beautiful day. Shafts of sunlight stream through the south-facing window, until one of the web developers pulls the blinds down ill-temperedly. I watch my screen, the emails dribbling in, the messages and requests from colleagues popping up as notifications. Already it seems strange that I had sat here, a week ago, two weeks ago, with a living, growing embryo inside me; such a thing seems to belong to the distant past, to another era entirely. Now there is only this: the road ahead. It is somehow both harder and easier to bear the weight of what's happened now that I know what to expect, what to pack in the bag I'll take to the hospital next week, what the waiting room looks like, what it feels like to come round from general anaesthetic, how long it will take to recover, move on, get back to almost-normal. Almost.

★

The day of the operation we arrive at the hospital weighed down by our knowledge, and by the bag I have brought, the two heavy books I couldn't decide between, the laptop, so that I can finish up some work while we wait, the phone charger, the dressing gown, the fleece-lined slippers. I have not had anything to eat or drink since the previous evening, and already I feel slightly distanced from myself.

In the waiting room we wait. A woman and a man shuffle in, take a seat in the corner, under a bulletin board advertising research studies, support groups, statistics. The woman is sobbing into the man's shoulder. He is making soothing gestures. Her voice rises sometimes so that a word meets me on the other side of the room – *can't, just, now, I* . . .

After about five minutes a doctor enters the room, crouches before them, speaks softly, and they go out again, the three of them. The woman is still crying, though the sobs are silent, incorporated into the movement of her body, her shoulders.

Later, after I have been seen by the sonographer, who confirms what we already know, that there is no heartbeat, no growth, and asks if we want an image of the scan (we don't), we return to the waiting room. The only open seats next to each other are the ones beneath the bulletin board, so we take them. In the opposite corner is a woman with her partner and her bag, slippers peeking out, a wary stare. She's come prepared, as I have. She knows the drill. We exchange glances that say, *we've been here before.* I see her again an hour later, when I'm done waiting in this room and am ready to wait in a new place, a small curtained-off area with a bed for me and a chair for Alexander, where doctors and nurses will come and take my vital signs and ask me questions and prep me for the operation. She's in the curtained-off area next to mine, sitting on the chair, her partner leaning on the bed, and our eyes meet again just before the curtain is pulled, and though our faces make no movement at all a perfectly shared moment of understanding passes between us, palpable to me, physically palpable.

When the nurse arrives to question us, to prepare us, the woman on the other side of the curtain echoes my responses. Yes, I've had this procedure before. Yes, it was done here. No, I'm not allergic to anything.

The nurse who leads me to theatre, in my slippers and my bathrobe to cover the open-arsed gown, is devastatingly beautiful. To put me at ease she talks to me more as if I'm a peer than a patient – because I've been here before, because I know where I'm going, because I've done everything right. What is it about moments of physical vulnerability that always make me want to be the *best*, the best at following the rules, at not troubling anyone? I want every medical professional I come into contact with to go away admiring me, admiring how well I play the role of patient, how intelligent and informed and yet also submissive I am. I lie and say to the nurse that I feel calmer because I know what to expect, willing it to be true, wanting to be brave for her, this lovely, beautiful woman, wanting her to prefer me to all the other patients she'll see today. 'That's interesting!' she says. 'There's another woman here who said she's more nervous than she was the first time.' I want immediately to rescind my statement, issue a new one: *me too!* But I can no longer remember what the truth is, whether I feel more or less nervous than I did the first time I shuffled down this hall. I hardly know what I feel, except sad. Sadder than before, I think – but then I wonder if this is just time playing tricks: how, after all, would you quantify this particular sadness, measure it up against other similar sadnesses? Why impose a hierarchy, when sadness itself adheres to no rules?

Still, it's hard not to think of the double life, the other track. The couple in the waiting room at the clinic, receiving their scan photo, all smiles at the start of a journey that ends not here but somewhere happier, or somewhere else, at least.

7

A Fear

A stillness, a silence, which is also a fear.

The fear is this: that I will never reproduce. That this will keep happening, again and again, even though, as I have often been told, it's statistically unlikely to, even though there's really no reason to think that it will, even though *at least I know I can get pregnant*, even though I'm *still so young*. I don't necessarily believe this will be my story, but it's impossible not to feel the threat of it.

Fear of never reproducing is, of course, somewhere deep down tied to a primal fear of disappearance, of extinction on both an individual and a grand scale. All this interest in genealogy lately, all these DNA tests, spitting into a plastic tube and mailing it off to a lab, receiving a report on your genetic make-up, at least in a geographical sense: isn't it about reaffirming our biological links? Isn't it about tracing back, as our ancestors will have imaginatively traced forward, the line of our existence?

My mother's mother was adopted. She was raised by a working-class American Jewish couple in Brooklyn, but her biological parents were Russian, also Jewish, immigrants. For a long time that's all anyone knew. But recently my uncle did some digging and discovered that they were both, the biological parents, institutionalised when their daughter was still a baby. The reasons cited for this are vague, but mental illness is indicated, and it's assumed that this is why their only child was given up for adoption. A break in the link. How do we account, in all these charts and trees, for such things – for breaks, anomalies?

I'm not as interested in my own family history as I should be, at least not in the abstract: I don't need to see a map that shows me that less than 1 per cent of my genetic material originates from the Iberian Peninsula. At the same time, yes, when I think about that stillness, that silence, what I see is it reverberating for generations. I see my own disappearance, a kind of slow fading away. This is not what I think makes a parent. It is not why I want to have a baby, or not only why. Certainly it is not the best thing (though also not the worst) I think I could give my child: my genes. But I cannot look through the tunnel and see my own prospective absence – my genealogical silence – and not wonder at it.

Is this selfish? Yes. It is selfish. But it is what I feel, a fear that is also a desire, a desire that is also a fear. If I had a baby in my arms right now, at this very moment, would it be any less selfish a desire? Would it be any less compelling?

I think of the scan photograph we were offered before the D&C, how quickly and decisively we said no. All I could think in the moment was that what I wanted to remember was *not this*. I don't regret that decision, not for a moment. On the other hand, tucking the photograph we *do* have away in a file, I wonder what traces of the experience, of my own memory, will remain. I don't particularly want to look at this image either, as it turns out, and yet I'm afraid of what will happen if I don't.

Rachel Cusk: *in terms of history silence was forgetting, and it was the one thing people feared most of all, when it was their own history that was at risk of being forgotten.*

★

When I was a child I read somewhere that death is when the heart stops beating. I worried, for a time, over the logistics of this: how, I wondered, did the heart know to go on beating?

What if it decided to stop before the rest of a body was ready for it to stop?

This puzzle returned to me later, as a teenager, during a particularly potent bout of anxiety, in the form of panic attacks. Every night for a month I lay in bed entirely unconvinced I would wake the next morning. There was nothing, so far as I knew, wrong with my heart, or with any other part of my body, but even after that month, sometimes I woke with my pulse racing, feeling nauseous and disorientated, and I was convinced, I was certain, that I was dying – if not immediately, in the moment, then certainly more slowly, from some invisible, undiagnosed, unlikely illness.

Listen to your body. A thing that people say. Yoga teachers, in their singsong voices, exhale the words as a kind of gentle warning: don't do anything you're not comfortable with. Don't feel you have to compare or compete. Listen to *your* body. Doctors, unsure how to treat you, what to treat you for, say it with trained concern: I want to take you seriously, but I can't know for sure what is going on in the hidden places, so listen to your body. Call if anything changes. But what am I listening for? I feel at odds with my body, as if there's something it's withholding from me. If I understand, intellectually, that it is folly to think this way – the mind is not some separate entity, the body is not the baser part of me – I also understand that living with the discrepancy between desire and *this, here, now* involves a process of continual re-evaluation of that most fundamental relationship, and this process involves a kind of fragmentation of self. The self I want to be – able to reproduce as effortlessly as it is ever possible for a human to reproduce – and the self I seem to be – a self to whom the process of reproduction is shrouded in some kind of mystery – are competing for my attention, and my trust. Which is the real issue: I want to listen to my body, of course, but how can I trust it, let alone understand it? A panic attack can feel like a heart attack, anxiety can manifest as illness, illness can go undetected; we can be utterly convinced of one thing when something else entirely is true. An embryo that is somehow both part of your body and entirely its own body can cease growing, and your body can do nothing about it, can *say* nothing about it.

In other words: all this time I've spent thinking about what the body *knows*, and really what I've been learning is what it *doesn't* know, or what it can't say. Straying further and further into the wilds of *here be dragons*, where there are a million what ifs. Chief among them: what if this is something my body *doesn't* know how to do? What if the knowledge, the ability, simply isn't there?

8

(())

My boss at the office gives me a few extra days off after the D&C. I'm grateful, though I'm not sure if I need them or not: by the end of the weekend I feel fine, physically, more or less, and home alone on Monday my skin crawls at the thought of all that time stretching out before me: the rest of the morning, the afternoon, the evening.

I arrange to meet a friend, but I cannot wait to get going, to get out, to be in the world again. I walk into town early, buy a guidebook to Portugal, where we're going on holiday with my parents next month. At a shop that I have always liked but never felt I could afford I buy a light cashmere jumper and a dress that even on sale is too expensive, but which I can picture myself wearing with flat leather sandals in Lisbon, sitting outside with a sweating glass of beer. I imagine what it will be like to be there, to touch the cold glass, to feel the dress brushing my calves, to put the jumper over my shoulders as evening falls.

My friend and I share a thick slice of lemon cake at a café in the centre of town. The magnolia trees are starting to blossom; it feels like the first day of the year in which not only spring but what will come after is palpable, is *happening*. I feel almost unconscionably cheerful: I have my new dress, my guide to Portugal, the sun is shining, there is nothing, for now, to be afraid of, my body is my own, who can tell the future? When I speak with my friend about the miscarriage I am able only to convey this sense of pragmatism and light-heartedness, even though I know, and she knows, that it isn't the whole picture.

After the cake my friend needs to run an errand on my side of the city, so we agree to walk together. Unexpectedly, as we are striding down the High Street, she mentions her own miscarriage. She has never spoken of it except that one time, years ago: another spring day, not entirely unlike this one, in fact, in the garden of her rented house, while we sipped dark beer and smoked the cigarettes she rolled. Her life now is almost unrecognisable to her life then – different partner, different home, different career – and yet the flash of familiarity momentarily dissolves these distinctions between *then* and *now*, between who we were and who we are, while also strangely solidifying them: here we are, among the blossoms again, different versions of ourselves. Speaking with her now it is clear that time has done what it always does to events which mark but do not define us; she misremembers details, getting wrong the year it happened, for example, then correcting herself as we collectively trace our shared history back. But these details, in a sense, though they mattered at the time, perhaps matter very little now.

My life would have looked so different, she says. Which is really, in the end, all you can say. *A double life.*

★

Writers and editors sometimes use the letters 'TK' to mark places in a manuscript where additional material is still to come, but I have taken instead to marking the places where I know I still have more to write, where I know the rhythm isn't yet right, where a word that I can't place yet is still missing, with a form of parentheses, a visualisation or manifestation of the gaps in my thoughts: (())

I do this partly because it seems that the space better represents the possibility inherent in what's still unfinished than a pair of letters could – but also, I realise now, because sometimes I am afraid to say the thing that fills the space.

Kate Zambreno: *Perhaps silence can actually be read as a form of writing, that recognizes language's failure, the impossibility and anemia of words.*

In the aftermath of the miscarriage, I find that words are not just anaemic but elusive. *Language is always late . . .* without it, until it comes, I have a series of gaps, of holes or spaces, which approximate silences. Even in my notebook, writing only for myself, I work continually *around* the thing that I mean; I cannot or will not name the miscarriage except as *this*, as if it were so self-evident as to need no name, or else as if it has no name. *I know that the underlying, deep sadness of now, this particular moment, weighs heavy, seeps into everything,* I write. *Nothing is untouched, and it's difficult to pick up on the nuances of doubt: what was there before? What's just an echo of this?* I have a sense of wanting to burn things down, start fresh – *fuck the job, fuck the PhD,* I write – but instead I make a list of tangible things to do for the future: people to talk to about freelance work, updates to make to my website, things to ask my PhD supervisor. And then one little bullet point at the end: *And there's the physical recovery, too: which will be a positive thing.*

What I mean by the physical recovery is: when I stop bleeding, when I stop cramping. When I can swim again, regain my strength, or at least my routine. But I think I also mean: a reconciliation. A restoration of trust. I want to feel a part of the world. I want to do as Nan Shepherd does, and lie down in this wilderness, and feel it in my arms, my legs, against my skin, know it by its taste and its smell, listen to its silence. If I could do that, could I also begin to correspond with it, and in that way with my body? What if I could unlearn, or unknow, the assumptions I've always had about my body, and start again, from a position of relative neutrality? A kind of faith, a re-inhabiting. *Slowly I have found my way in.*

Yes: in a month there I'll be, in Portugal, the beer, the breeze, the dress, my skin warm after a day in the sunshine. In the western Algarve we'll walk for miles along the edge of the country, to a windy point from where we will watch huge waves rolling in, waves so large they are hard to fathom. The wind will be so loud it will drown out all other sound, all conversation. Later we'll find a beach from which to jump into an unfamiliar ocean; my hair will smell of salt, my flipflops will slap against the rough bottoms of my feet on the way back to the car. On our last night before flying home Alexander and I will sit outside in a square in Lisbon, drinking wine from a kiosk café, the air soft despite the late hour. Cigarette smoke will drift towards us, children's voices, the sound of bells somewhere. The wine will be sweet.

Of course it's never that simple, is it? To reconcile with the body, to correspond with it, requires being attentive not only to the *pleasures of Sensation* but also to the fury that's growing like a weed, to the anger held and withheld. You have to find and feel the places where that anger has settled, hear even what you do not want to hear. I will learn this, too, in time. But you have to start somewhere, don't you – and why not with a roaring wind, the smell of salt, the sweetness of the wine, the softness of the air?

Four

The Canyon

2016

I

The Disappearance

Spring, and everyone is pregnant. The writer I follow on Twitter, the schoolmate on Facebook, the friend of a friend at a dinner party who delicately declines the homemade chocolate mousse even though the NHS guidelines on eggs are clear, 'just to be on the safe side'. The woman on TV, the woman on the bus, the woman in the waiting room, the woman in the pub, the woman from the pool, the one with the pink cap and the blue costume, who stops swimming for a while and then reappears suddenly, her belly small but distinctly round, telling a friend, 'it's a boy!'

Maybe it's just the season, the way the blossom dripping from the magnolia trees resembles something fleshly, erotic, the way fallow ground is suddenly bursting forth with wood anemones and alliums and wild sweet peas, the way the air feels moist in a way that promises life, like a kiss – but it seems to me an epidemic of catastrophic proportions. Is no one else worried? Where did they all find the time to have so much sex? Christ, I think, does the world really need that *many* more people? Couldn't they at least pace themselves a little, stagger it? What will happen to the workforce in a few months' time? Do they have to rub their bellies in so self-satisfied a way, unconsciously, maliciously, as they talk to me, as they wait to be seated at a restaurant, as they cross the road?

Uncharitable, true. Unfair. A gross exaggeration. But still.

What if the thing I crave is not just pregnancy itself but the *visibility* of a pregnant body? The way people notice you, see you, pay attention to you. Even though often, I know, that attention is unwelcome, inappropriate: strangers reaching out, touching a stomach they have no claim over, policing consumption of coffee or wine, playing the role of a benevolent authority even if they would not, when it came down to it, give up their seat on the Tube.

But the thing I feel is that without this, you could just disappear. As a person, and as a woman particularly. Walking down the street, dodging other pedestrians, flattening yourself against a wall so that a buggy can pass unimpeded, or folding into yourself on the subway next to a sprawling man, making yourself smaller and smaller until . . . nothing remains. Which of course is the opposite of a healthy pregnancy, during which your body grows and grows until it doesn't resemble itself, until it becomes unignorable, until . . . something emerges. Until new life, in more ways than one.

I worry that I am disappearing, eroding, failing, writes the author Emilie Pine of what she calls her 'baby years', the years of trying and miscarrying and hoping and despairing. *I only want to be a mother,* she writes. *Why is it so easy for some people and so hard for others? Why is it so hard for me?* I read and reread that last sentence, each time with a different emphasis, a different urgency. Why *is* it so hard for me? *Why* is it so hard for me? Finally, most selfishly, most pressingly: why is it so hard for *me*?

I too worry that I am disappearing. At parties and gatherings I am increasingly convinced no one can see me. People look past me as I'm talking to them, or bump into me as if I am not there. They ask me the same question twice, do not remember my answer. They introduce themselves to me even though we have met already, even though we have met several times already. They get my name wrong, and I do not correct them. I resent this, but I also feel that to some extent I understand it, that to some extent I deserve it. I know I have become boring, I have become flimsy, because I can only think of one thing, of a lack, an empty space, about which there is nothing to say to strangers, nothing to be said. I have in a sense *become* the empty space. I stick to safe, dull topics: how my thesis is progressing (slowly), how much it's rained recently (a lot). And who ever remembers the mousy woman at the dinner party who spoke only, and briefly, of the weather?

What would it mean, I sometimes wonder, to insert something unignorable into the space between us – the swoop and arc of a large belly, the conspicuousness of it, a whole future not quite hidden under stretched skin? The *normalcy* of it, the quiet heroism of it. I think of Maggie Nelson describing being saluted by members of the armed services in the airport during her pregnancy. Even if all you are doing is waiting for your flight to be called, you are Important. You have a presence.

I know that it is not this simple, of course. I know that motherhood can be its own kind of disappearance, or else an uncomfortable exhibition – shortly after the anecdote about being saluted Nelson writes for example of how *the pregnant body in public is also obscene*; we revere it in the abstract, but fear its actual messy materiality, the way it externalises internal processes and desires. I know too that what I'm asking for is its own kind of curse, a regressive, destructive desire to be seen purely in terms of my own biological function – but in these moments of short-sightedness my imagination fails me, and in the murk I can perceive only the outline of a terrifying private fear, which I can't look quite in the face, but which I feel like a shadow: that without a child, without a visible, tangible pregnancy, I am nothing, no one, invisible.

If I think about my situation logically, this fear makes no sense, not least because when I look at the lives of the women I know without babies I don't think they are *nothing*, far from it. I don't think that a person has to be a parent to live a valuable life, to find meaning and form, to contribute something (and what does that mean anyhow, 'to contribute'?). And yet if I'm honest, brutally honest with myself, I am not sure I can yet do myself the same courtesy that I do others, not sure that I can yet see myself as a *person* independent of my reproductive history or potential. In fact what I have felt with each miscarriage is the slipping away of a chance at what if I had to name it I would call A Real Life – a real life not only for the collection of cells that was never a baby, but also for myself, for my husband. A life with substance.

I think I have felt for some time now that we are simply floating along, waiting for something to begin, for the outlines of our life to solidify. I guess if I think about our life now what I see is something fuzzy, without definition, something that I don't know how to shape, or to grab on to. I see us wandering, together but also slightly apart, through a landscape I still don't quite know how to describe except to say what it lacks, what it isn't.

It isn't littered with our child's toys, it isn't baby-proofed, it isn't breathlessly busy days and sweetly sleepless nights. It isn't what I expected.

*

One day, in early spring, a few weeks after the second miscarriage, I found myself on the bus. I had recovered, physically at least. I was on my way to work. Outside it was raining, hard, relentlessly, and inside the windows were steamed up, so that my impression of the world going by was clouded by other people's breath. I was soaked to the skin from waiting for the bus, my face hot and cold at the same time, and for no specific reason, but lots of little ones, my eyes were blurred with tears.

It seemed to me in this moment that the weight of an unspecific sadness might eventually make it impossible to breathe, impossible to sleep, to eat, to work. It might in fact dissolve all notions of *me*, *I*, leaving just the outline of something, a puddle on a seat. I did not actually feel myself at imminent risk of this; I felt just the threat of it, like a stranger's breath on my neck, raising my hackles. It *could* happen. If. If what? If I stayed here, in this place, this landscape of almost-motherhood, of maybe-maybe-not.

For a wild moment I contemplated the possibility that some drastic change, some deviation, might be the only way forward – why, for example, was I on a bus at all, running late for a job I felt no passion for, wearing a pair of shoes that were an awkward compromise between practical and professional, carrying a broken umbrella? Why was I in this city, of all the cities in the world? What in fact was stopping me from – I don't know, from dyeing my hair red, from booking a ticket to Paris or Istanbul, from starting over, from turning around right now and going home and calling Alexander and saying: let's get out of here?

But I stayed on the bus. I got off at my stop. I swiped my key card at reception, walked upstairs, sat at my desk, turned my computer on, made a cup of instant coffee, watched the emails roll in. And while I stirred the Nescafé granules into my mug I told myself to remember a simple fact: that after the first miscarriage I had been sad for a while, too, but also that, after a period of time, that sadness had been incorporated into my body, and I was not sad anymore, except in an abstract, retrospective way. I told myself that this would happen again, and this knowledge was in itself a form of solace; I would not dissolve; I could speak to myself through the lens of my own experience, and trust the source. I had no reason to lie to myself.

I was, as it turns out, right to trust myself, right to trust that this would happen again. An invisible line: before, I was viscerally sad, and now, I am not, or not in the same way, at least. But this time I find that the sadness has not been incorporated into my body so much as consumed by something, something big and mean: a kind of rage, an ugliness, a twisted growth with offshoots of envy, resentment, self-loathing. I find it harder and harder, as the spring progresses, to stifle even the foulest feelings about myself, and about others. I think, often and irrationally:

they have something I want. Or else, simply: *I want.* I lack. I see a canyon, and the canyon is both inside me, and between me and the rest of the world. I think in other words of *us* and *them*, except the *us* is always just *I*, except the *them* is everyone else.

Is my marriage in a good place? Are my friendships? My relationship with my family, with my husband's family? I don't know. Maybe, maybe not. Certainly there's a limited language with which to express what to me is so self-evident – that I have failed (again!) at something essential – and I suspect that if I were to try to say this with true honesty, without softening the blow, without acknowledging again that yes, I'm still young, that no, there's no reason to believe it won't happen someday, that in many ways I am lucky, in many ways I am in a position of exceptional privilege, I would find myself alienated, alone. In any case Alexander is often at work, and I am often angry not at him but at the world in a way that in turn makes him angry; underlying nearly every conversation we have is my own inarticulable resentment of myself, which frequently comes out as resentment of others, him included. There is only so much he can do or say to ease what feels to me an unequal burden: the failure, it seems, is mine and mine alone, and so I must bear its consequences alone, even though – or perhaps precisely because – they are consequences that impact us both. In moments of particular despair I look at him and I think: why should he have to stay here, in this place, in this marriage, when we know the problem isn't his, we know his sperm are perfectly capable?

In truth I have often thought about what it means for our extended families, this thing, this unidentified issue, this will-we-won't-we maybe-maybe-not whirlpool we're spinning in. I am an only child. Alexander's brothers are nine years younger, and they are both gay, which means that when – if – they decide to have children, it will be complicated, biologically at least, from the start. We do not have the consolation of nieces and nephews, not yet, maybe not ever. Our parents do not have other grandchildren to look to. I think sometimes of the kindness Alexander's parents have shown me, by not being resentful, not being impatient. Do they ever look at their eldest son and think: *if only he had struck up a conversation with someone else that night?* They might have multiple grandchildren by now if he had, if instead of me he had met some other woman, with a more obedient body, a more forthcoming womb. *I* certainly do: I look at him and I think that he might be a father already if not for me, that the only thing standing in his way is bad luck, or something in the shadow-parts of me that neither of us can see, that not even the doctors can see. I think, as many people do about their partners, that he would be, will be, a truly wonderful parent, and it seems during my darker forays along this line of thought that I have somehow deprived him of this opportunity.

In anger, in spite, I have once or twice said to him that he ought to leave, or at least ought to feel free to. Find a woman for whom this is easier. *A real woman*, I have said. *Get on with your life.* Maybe I have even meant it, in the moment. Maybe I have even wanted it. I cannot escape the whims of my own body: he can.

My friends, meanwhile, are busy living their lives. I do not often contact them, at least partly because I am worried that if I hear one more platitude, one more conciliatory word, I will snap, I will say things I mean only in the heat of the moment, and not in that deeper part of myself that knows how irrational it is. *I will not be young forever, it does not help me to know that technically I can conceive, it is not a comfort to hear about your aunt's sister-in-law's cousin who had a miscarriage and went on to bear six healthy children.* The starker subtext: *I resent you, I reject your comfort, kindly as it's meant, because it doesn't match the pitch of my own anger, I would rather languish here alone than even look at you.*

If I look closely in the mirror I can see that I do not like the person I have become, or perhaps always was. I do not *want* to roll my eyes at every ultrasound image posted on Facebook, every twee announcement – a heart drawn in the sand, a hand-made T-shirt, a dog posed next to a chalkboard sign – and feel it like a stab in the chest. I do not want to hate, actually *hate* at times, perfect strangers, who bear me no ill will, who do not – and again perhaps this is the very problem – even seem to notice me. I do not want to zoom in on Instagram photos, looking for the beginnings of a bump, to read too much into every drink declined, to parse every sentence for clues, to feel heavy with perpetual dread that someone I care about, someone for whom I should be happy, is on the cusp of revealing a pregnancy – and yet I do, I am, I can't help it.

I wonder sometimes what it would be like to feel nothing but uncomplicated joy every time an acquaintance or a relative or a celebrity reveals that they're pregnant. What would it take to overcome my self-obsession, to see beyond or, better yet, entirely independently of, my own uncertain relationship with reproduction? Perhaps if I could do this I could also somehow forgive myself for a failure and a lack that, logically, I know I have no control over.

But then again: does anybody feel that way all the time? Happiness and nothing more, no little niggle of self-doubt or self-destructive hostility, no envy, no judgement, never, nowhere, not even deep down in the inaccessible places?

★

I suppose what I mean when I say I have been waiting for A Real Life to begin is this: I have been deferring all decisions except the Big One, the one we made almost three years ago. And it feels now as if we are slipping off the map of our own future. All around us everyone seems to be moving perpet-ually forwards: they are changing jobs, getting promotions, somehow, miraculously, buying houses and flats and doing them up, extending kitchens and converting lofts, contributing to pensions, publishing books, starting businesses, adopting pets, posting idyllic photos of expensive-looking holidays on

Instagram, marrying, divorcing, moving to new cities. And, yes: having babies. Going out less, or not at all; heading home early from the pub, declining another pint, looking ruefully, hungrily, at us, with our carefree life, as they depart. And we are still here: exactly where we were last year, the year before that, the year before that, the year before that . . .

We have put everything on hold. We did not mean to. We did not even realise we were doing it. But the kinds of questions you might ask of a marriage, of a shared life, cannot now be answered *until*. What is our future together going to look like? Where will we live? What will we do? What do we want, except this one fragile thing that may or may not come? We talk abstractly about the possibility of moving to California, finding a way to live on the ranch; we work out budgets, how much income we would need, how much time for Alexander to apply for a green card, how we would deal with the thorny issue of health insurance. But we cannot commit to the idea, cannot even seriously consider it, *until*. Neither of course can we commit to staying here in Oxford permanently, at least not *until* . . . There is no point in me trying to focus on a career when at any moment it might – but might not – be interrupted. Alexander certainly can't contemplate whether the job he is doing is in fact the one he wants to be doing *until*, not when we rely so heavily on the regularity of his salary, on the paid holiday time, the promise of paternity leave. Even travel plans must be weighed up against the uncertainty of *until*: where can we go that will still be feasible, still be safe, even if . . . ? Can we accept that invitation to a wedding in California? Can we visit that friend in Copenhagen later this year? Perhaps best not to commit, or at least to leave ourselves the option of backing out. Just in case.

What kind of relationship is this, then, when we cannot move forward, but also cannot take back the decision we've already made? The way we are with each other is somehow dependent on an outcome that neither of us can guarantee.

Still, we seem always to be saying. We'll live this way for now, just for now, until. *Until.* The problem being, of course, that there may never be an *until.* We may never reach that place; it may not exist for us. We live perpetually in the meanwhile – and meanwhile I can feel myself fading.

2

Incognito

All in all it's a blurry spring – the tears, the rain. Sometimes in England, particularly in the first half of the year, I feel that you could just wash away, like a chalk drawing on a sidewalk. I cycle to the pool on mornings that smell green and wet, sweating under my waterproof jacket. I peel my soaked jeans from my skin in the changing room. I listen to the conversations between two women who I often see getting dressed as I arrive. They always sound tired: their jobs are difficult, their husbands are difficult, their children cause them concern. One of them is very tall, with a thick tattoo that covers most of her left calf and another in the small of her back; the other is very short, with dyed blonde hair. Their lives do not sound enviable to me, but they sound solid, and as I listen to them I have that dissolving feeling, that chalk-on-a-sidewalk feeling. Routine, habit, gives me a sense of my own physical presence, but I wonder too if it contributes to my translucence, if the problem is that in doing the same things over and over again, visiting the same places, I have become part of the scenery myself. When I go to the pool, when I strip naked after a swim and stand under the showers in the changing room, I feel as invisible as if I were not there at all, as if I have no substance, although I am so close to the other naked bodies that I could reach out and touch them, so close that I see what few others do – the tattoo in the small of the tall woman's back, for instance, so intimate a piece of knowledge, the scars and marks, the bumps and folds.

The two women always finish dressing just as I finish undressing, and I always, in that moment, feel keenly both the impotence and the compulsion of habit. We do this dance every morning. What good does it do me? And yet I go, again and again.

No one knows me here, I think, with something like anger, with something like relief.

★

The German academic Christoph Heyl has written interestingly about the history of privacy. He describes, for example, a kind of black half-mask popular among well-off women in London in the seventeenth century. These masks were worn in part for protection – so that, as a poem by Charles Cotton put it, a woman might *save her beauty from the Air, / And guard her pale Complexion* – but also in part to disguise the wearer. Such a disguise was more notional than literal, since the masks covered only the upper half of the face. And yet, Heyl notes, this coverage was enough to *imply* concealment, and thus to allow the wearer, in a sense, to disappear. *These masks,* he writes, *offered new possibilities of playing with anonymity, and they probably gave a sense of protection, a sense of almost being invisible.* As appreciation for the anonymity a mask could confer on its wearer grew, other patterns of behaviour shifted in parallel. Eye contact between strangers, for example, became increasingly taboo; an author of a list of 'rules of behaviour' in *London Magazine* in 1734 advised readers *Not to fasten your Eyes upon any Person entering into a publick Room, for Fear . . . of shocking his Modesty.* The worry was in part that by meeting someone's eyes you could 'read' their face, and so interpret private or distasteful emotions: desire, say, or jealousy.

When I read this I think of the goggles I wear when I swim: the tightness of them, the coloured lenses, the way they mask my eyes but afford me clarity underwater. They do produce a sense of almost being invisible, even if it's a false sense: everyone at the pool is complicit in a kind of communal delusion of anonymity, I think, akin perhaps to the 'incognito ritual' Heyl describes, a sort of virtual form of disguise whereby *[i]f you made it understood that you were incognito, people could of course still recognise you, but they were nevertheless expected to behave towards you as if you were completely disguised.* I am under no illusion that my goggles, small and transparent as they are, obscure my identity, that, in my swimming costume, I will not one morning be recognised by somebody from a completely other facet of my life, or that I will not somehow give myself away just because I am more or less 'incognito'. But it is surely a form of playing with anonymity, a form of protection: *no one knows me here.* If no one can meet my eyes, perhaps they can't read the desire, the jealousy.

I think often these days about the freedom of that, but also the fear – that if no one knows me, perhaps I cannot be seen at all, perhaps the edges of what is possible will recede, or dissolve. I wake imagining the day ahead as a performance of sorts, an attempt to hide myself, to reveal myself, in equal measure. The pool is an essential part of this, because it allows me to imagine, and to project, a version of myself stripped of any but the most immediate physical histories. Yes, I have a bruise on my thigh where I walked into the edge of the bed yesterday, but no, you cannot see into me, into the empty spaces, into the uncharted depths.

I like stripping down in the changing room; I like the symbolism of it; I have never felt self-conscious standing there naked, applying deodorant, brushing my hair, while other women mill around, because I don't believe that in that state anything can be given away. The perfect mask, in a sense, is none at all. I have always, in that vein, appreciated the closeness between underwear and swimwear. When it comes down to it I communicate more through the rhythm of my stroke than the topography of my skin.

And yet the truth is more complicated. Isn't it always? The truth is that I want both: to be seen, acknowledged, and to hide, to disappear into the crowd. An impossible desire, but that can't be helped. Sometimes we simply want in too many directions at once.

3

The Uncharted Interior

The consultant I saw when I was miscarrying has scheduled me for an MRI, to map the shape of my uterus once and for all. We know from ultrasounds that it's what's known as bicornuate, heart-shaped, where the uterus is divided into two horns, but she would like to get a clearer picture than an ultrasound can give, to understand the extent of the division. It's unlikely, the consultant has stressed, that the shape of my uterus is a contributing factor to either my miscarriages or the difficulty I've had getting pregnant in the first place, but it's worth knowing, worth seeing inside, since we can. I suspect that she may be saying this simply to give me the illusion of progress, the illusion of control over my situation, but at the same time, I don't care: I'll take the illusion.

I have never had an MRI. I don't know what to expect except that it will be loud and I will have to lie very still for a long time while the images are captured. I find in the days preceding the procedure that I am actually looking forward to it, because I am tired, and the idea of lying down with my eyes closed for half an hour sounds relaxing.

The MRI department is located in a part of the hospital complex we have never visited, and Alexander and I get lost trying to find it. Finally we find that we are stuck in a full, staff-only car park shouting at each other. My appointment is in minutes. I can see the entrance to the MRI department from the car, though we cannot leave the car here without risking it being towed away or ticketed, so eventually I get out, slam the door. I do not kiss Alexander goodbye, or tell him that I love him, or tell him where to meet me later. I do not know how long I'll be – the letter I've received from the hospital is ambiguous. He offers to come and find me after he's located somewhere to park. There's no point, I say, just go and get a coffee somewhere, I'll call you when I'm done, I'll come to you. In that moment I am glad to be rid of him, of the car, of the need to arrange a rendezvous, of the need to hold someone's hand or worry about where they are going to sit when I am placed in the machine. Later I'll realise that I'm simply nervous, that the idea of someone seeing inside my body not only intimidates me but has activated a latent fear of discovery, of diagnosis, but now I only march away without looking back, pulling my jacket on, digging into my handbag for my appointment letter.

Inside the receptionist takes my letter and shows me to a small changing cubicle. She asks me to remove any jewellery, any clothing with metal zips or fasteners. My valuables, she says, can be placed in a locker. Into the locker I relinquish my phone, my wallet, my wedding ring. I take off my underwire bra, my jeans, pull on a pair of leggings. Then, thus attired, I sit and wait. Nearby a woman lies on a gurney, holding the hand of a man who stands beside her, and I avert my eyes. A child fiddles with the edge of a hospital gown while his mother taps something into her phone. A nurse calls my name and I follow her into a room, sit obediently on a bed while she asks me a series of questions and then, unexpectedly, tries to insert a cannula into a vein in my left hand. I did not realise there would be a cannula involved, or a drug administered intravenously. I feel my pulse quicken; I suddenly understand that I have come unprepared, emotionally if not physically. The nurse takes a few unsuccessful stabs at my vein, then apologises and summons a colleague to do it for her.

The drug, they say, will slow the movement of my bowels, so that they don't interfere with the image. It may also temporarily make my mouth dry and my vision blurry, so they hope I have someone to drive me home. I do, I say, and I wish suddenly that I had said yes, park and then come and find me, or at least that I hadn't shouted, that I hadn't slammed the door. They lead me into the room with the machine and I lie down, feet facing the entrance. The machine is small; I don't know what I was expecting, but somehow the smallness of it seems impossible, surely my body cannot fit in there. I am issued with headphones, which will block out some of the noise of the machine and through which someone will communicate with me at regular intervals to give me instructions. They place a panic button near my right index finger. I feel, or imagine, the coldness of the bowel-slowing drug entering my vein. 'If you feel unwell or want to be pulled out,' someone says, 'press the button,' but they are saying this *as* the machine is sucking me in, as first my feet, then my torso, then my head are swallowed up: it is too late for me to absorb what is happening, what they are saying. Too late for me to realise that I don't want to be here.

I have never considered myself claustrophobic, but now I open my eyes to discover that the ceiling of the machine is pressing down on my gaze, that the whole weight of the world is drumming into me. It's not that I'm not claustrophobic, I realise, but simply that I have never before been in a space small enough to spark the feeling. I am immediately dizzy, and my pulse feels far too fast, too erratic, but it is even worse if I close my eyes, even though they have told me that I might find the experience more relaxing with my eyes closed, so there I lie, staring at the ceiling, wondering if this constitutes panic, if I would be warranted in using the button. For a while I cannot stop myself from shaking, which is counter to the goal of complete stillness. Does *that* constitute a reason to use the button? I wish again that I had not been so uncharitable to my husband, who otherwise might be, if not *here* with me, then at least reassuringly in a room nearby. I regret that we fought about nothing, or anything: who cares whose fault it was that we turned left when we should have gone right?

Eventually I play a game with myself: I go through the alphabet, A to Z, and list a different name for each letter. *Alfred, Beatrice, Catriona, David* . . . When I reach Q and I can think of nothing I give myself permission to skip it. When I reach *Zelda* I start again, trying not to repeat any names. Why this soothes me I don't know, but eventually I decide that enough time has elapsed that it would be stupid to press the button now: the scan has already begun, data is being collected, and anyway I would only have to re-enter the tube at some point.

Somewhere out there, I imagine, a technician is pressing buttons, operating the machine, gathering the necessary images. I do not know if this is how it works, but I imagine that these images come up on a screen in real time, that the technician is looking through me now, as I lie here, and the awareness of this possibility makes my body feel both more and less solid.

After the MRI Alexander and I make up without really making up: no one apologises, no one really remembers what we were fighting about, no one cares. We have a pint at the pub at the end of our road and I tell everyone we run into, breathlessly, that I've just had an MRI, that it turns out I'm more claustrophobic than I thought. 'What a time to discover that!' I say, like it has been an adventure, which in a way I suppose it has. Then we go home and make dinner, and things go back to normal, to routine, to the way they are. In a month or two the consultant will call: nothing about the images they've gathered indicates that the shape of my uterus should be a particular hindrance to either conception or pregnancy.

I cannot see what she sees; the images are of me, but not for me, they would, I'm sure, not be legible even if they were laid out in front of me. But as she speaks to me I will think, briefly, of what she is seeing, of how she is able to interpret the imagery; of how, in fact, she is probably seeing me more clearly than anyone ever has before, if seeing me means seeing *inside me*, into the deepest parts, the uncharted interior – and of how, even then, with all that vision, there's still so little to tell, so little that can be known.

4

Onion

A fixation: I cannot seem to get the woman at the pool with the pink cap, the blue costume and the burgeoning belly out of my head.

I don't know her. I know her stroke, true, that she swims slightly slower than I do, but more aggressively, that she will not, for example, pause at the wall to even out a speed discrepancy but will plough on regardless, even if it means she has to pass someone at an inopportune moment, or that she is holding someone up. (I resent this, but I also on some level envy it: the audacity, the solidness of it – the way it seems to say unapologetically, *I am here*; I on the other hand am often so anxious to get out of other people's way that I only make things worse.) I know she has thick hair, that she is tall, that she takes long showers after she swims. But when I think of her she has no name, her face is a blank, and I feel a chill grip my head and my guts, a momentary loss of control that I recognise, without fully understanding it, as *envy*.

I hate myself for it, but I cannot abandon the obsession. Will there ever come a point, I wonder, when my first thought on seeing her with her growing belly isn't: *that should be me*? Because it should, I think. It would be, if things were different, if I hadn't miscarried, if, if, if.

Here's another thing I almost-know about her: once I saw her kiss a man in the shallow end of the medium lane. He was naked from the waist up, in baggy trunks, and as they embraced

I could almost feel the clamminess of the close wet skin, the cold rubbery surface of it. I think it was the first time I had ever seen two people kissing like that in the pool, as if they were not being observed, as if there, in the same lane, were not people chugging up and down, counting out lengths before work. As if they were on holiday, or on the street, or in the pub.

Is he the father? I wonder now.

I think about the reason this image has stayed with me: because it hints at a life outside the pool. When I think of that kiss, I think of the way it disrupts the neatness of the division between *out there* and *in here*. Of the way it makes a mockery of lines – there is no out there, no in here, no way to cross something that doesn't exist. And when I think of the hump of her belly I see how impossible it is to maintain that division, to separate oneself into swimmer on the one hand and woman on the other, and how maybe it would be easier, better, to stop trying so hard to maintain this kind of rigid division.

The anthropologist Mary Douglas once argued that we all have two bodies, a physical body and a social body. The social body, she says, *constrains the way the physical body is perceived.* Others, such as the scholar and novelist John Harvey, have expanded on this idea, suggesting that, for example, we have several different social bodies, which correspond to different social contexts (the 'beach body', the 'bedroom body', the 'smart body'). When we clothe ourselves it is partly to suggest, or to create, the body we are inhabiting: we do not, generally speaking, wear a bikini to the office, or a pantsuit to the beach, which, according to Harvey, *perhaps means that the body that is shown or hidden in smart clothes is not the same body that is shown openly for all to see in beachwear.* But what if – when – our bodies start to bleed together? What if the separation dissolves? The anthropologist Daniel Miller has written against the idea that we all have a real or essential 'self' hidden within us, beneath the layers of clothing and behaviour that signify social or cultural meaning. It is easy to imagine that by peeling away the layers, we might at some point get to the crux, the core, the single truth. *The* body, to adapt Douglas's and Harvey's parlance. And yet, Miller concludes, such a self does not exist: *we are all onions. If you keep peeling off our layers you would find – absolutely nothing left.*

If I am trying, in other words, to hide myself at the pool, or if I am imagining that somewhere deep down, somewhere that an MRI or a blood test might eventually reveal, is a kernel of irrefutable truth that will suddenly make sense of everything – then I am mistaken. My goggles are no mask, my costume is no armour, and my transparency is no indication of anything. I'll be hiding forever, seeking forever, if I go on like this.

*

A few years ago, I had just finished a swim when a woman I recognised – tall, about my age, a much stronger and faster swimmer than me but with a particularly unsociable backstroke – hurried up to me in the changing room. She knew it was a strange request, she said, but she wondered if she could use my phone for a moment. She spoke quickly, breathlessly: she had, she said, just started her swim when suddenly it struck her that perhaps she was meant to be elsewhere.

'I have a feeling,' she said, 'that I'm supposed to be at a physio appointment right now. I just need to check my email quickly, but I don't have a signal.'

'Of course,' I said, fishing in my bag for my phone. She dried her hands on her towel and took it from me; a few moments later she handed it back.

'I knew it,' she said, already pulling her swimsuit off, reaching for her T-shirt, 'shit!' She had to rush off, she went on – she'd let me log her out, she trusted me, she said, I remember that very specifically, because as far as I was concerned she had no good reason to, and yet I think I would have felt the same: the levelling, democratising influence of the pool, the costume, the near-nakedness, the intimacy, the anonymity. She was gone before I could even promise to do as she asked.

Later, after my shower, I looked at my phone. She had left the browser window with her email open. Visible was a folder labelled 'Emails from my ex'. I thought for a moment about this: about what it would mean to have such a folder, what it would mean to have such trust in a stranger not to look at it. I thought particularly about the story I could almost but not quite see, about the life that was almost visible, almost perceptible, like a mountain shrouded in mist. I thought about how often I had seen this woman, and known nothing more about her than her speed relative to mine in the pool. And so now what did I know? Nothing, or everything. That she was human, that she had a life beyond these walls, a past, a future, an ex whose emails she had kept for sentimental reasons, or legal reasons, or no good reason at all.

I thought for a long while about clicking on the folder, reading the emails, or at least one of them, just to get a flavour of the situation, just to peek, to learn a little more. But instead I logged out, closed the tab, cycled home: better perhaps not to know, better for this woman to remain to me an outline only, for anonymity – hers, mine – to be preserved.

5

The Announcement

One night, Alexander comes home from work. A colleague has just announced that she is pregnant. He is upset. I have never seen him like this; this is usually my territory – the rage, the envy, the irrationality of a response you have no control over. How often has he said to me, in sympathy, in frustration: there's no point getting angry about it?

Now he says: I know it's irrational, but I can't help it.

Another person's pregnancy can feel like the loss of yours – however theoretical your own pregnancy may have been, writes the journalist Nell Frizzell, which is maybe exactly what it feels like. And of course in this case it isn't theoretical at all, is it? I suggest to Alexander that perhaps it's hit so hard because his colleague's due date is close to when mine would have been had I not miscarried, that this is around the time we, too, could have been announcing a pregnancy. At first he quibbles with the comparison – her due date isn't the same, he says; well, close enough, I say, it's within a few weeks of mine – then he denies the whole thing: it's nothing to do with that, he says hotly, as if I'm being crazy.

He cooks steaks for dinner, with a salad and a Béarnaise sauce. The steaks are slightly overdone and he is furious with himself for the mistake, inconsolably so. The evening, soured already, is spoiled. I slap plates on the table so hard they rattle.

He pours the wine resentfully and messily; a bright red drop runs down the edge of my glass. We eat in sullen, angry silence. We say nothing for the rest of the meal. We say nothing, later, about the incident at all.

6

A Natural

At work I am responsible for helping to organise a social event for the office – a picnic in the park, sunshine, coolers full of beer, partners and children welcome. I am an anomaly in the company: the only female employee, and one of few without children. At the picnic the wives seem to form a cluster, even though many of them have never met before; they drink soda while their children clamp round their legs. One colleague's wife has just had their second child, a little boy; she holds him in a sling and he sleeps soundly through most of the afternoon. When he wakes up, he is passed around ritually among the other women. One of them, newly married, is praised particularly for the way she holds him. *A natural.* Someone looks at her husband, a glint in her eyes. *I'm seeing a baby in your future,* she says playfully. (She is right: less than a year later they will be expecting their first child.) I am pointedly not handed the baby, not even briefly, not even when I am closest to the mother and she needs to give him to someone so that she can take her turn at boules. I have never been called *a natural.*

I think: *they can see. They can tell.* I think I must give off a smell, a whiff of desperation, of unmotherliness. I swallow a sip of warm canned lager. I hate them; I want to be them.

7

Want

At university I dated a boy from Boston, where we were both studying. It was a serious relationship, and sometimes on cold winter afternoons we would walk down Commonwealth Avenue and imagine ourselves in one of the townhouses into whose windows we could tantalisingly glance: glimpses of Christmas trees, mirrors, dining tables, paintings, bookcases, someone sipping a glass of something that sparkled in the right light. We began to sketch something like a future together, although it was very aspirational; we never discussed exactly what we would do next summer, or next year, or when we graduated, it was always *someday*. Someday a townhouse like this one, someday a car like that one, a grand piano, a flatscreen TV, annual vacations in hot places with pools and tennis courts.

I was seduced by this image of myself living an ostentatious East Coast capitalist life, this image of myself as a polished professional woman, a career in law or politics, an assistant, a BlackBerry, very shiny hair, very high heels. But whenever we speculated about the future, our future, even though we sometimes touched on things like marriage, we never discussed – and I never imagined – having children. And no wonder: we were so young! But when I met Alexander, I was also very young still, and within a month or so of knowing him I began to feel that I wanted to have children with him – not then, not immediately, but certainly, if we stayed together, someday. It was a conviction that seemed to come out of nowhere, and it surprised me utterly.

I had never thought before about the emotional pull, let alone the mechanics, of having children, except in negative terms: in college once, my period a week late, I had mused on how unready I was even to contemplate a pregnancy, my mind made up about what I would do even before I took the test (negative); I had always been prissy and fastidious about birth control, had always seen myself as someone who would get all her ducks in a row first – the career, the house, the car, the vacations by the pool.

Where had this conviction come from, then? Was it a desire that had always been there, latent, or did it have to be created by something – some circumstance, a spark? But it turned, over the years, into an active aspiration, an *I want*. It built itself up, it took on a life of its own. It was something about which we unequivocally agreed. And when I say, now, that I feel the edges of our Real Life dissolving, what I am saying is that I put too much stock in the idea that simply to want is, eventually, to have. I invested in the fantasy on the assumption that it was, if not exactly a safe bet, then also not exactly an unlikely outcome.

Tracing the origin of a desire like *children* is futile: is it biological, an evolutionary impulse, a culturally imposed aspiration? But when I think about where it emerged, for me, I think about a particular weekend, very early on in my relationship with Alexander. We'd been invited to babysit for Alexander's boss and his wife, who had three boys, aged six, eight and ten. After their parents had left for the evening we played football with the boys in the summer evening light, and then we made pizzas and watched a bit of TV and told them now it was time to brush their teeth and go to bed, and finally we read a chapter of Harry Potter to them, putting on silly voices. I had never really done things like that before with children and it had never occurred to me except abstractly that there could be pleasure in it, but there was. I was scared, too, because I didn't know the family very well yet, and I didn't know how to talk to or look after children, really, and in many ways I was still a child myself – but seeing Alexander with them made plain to me that somehow, someday, together, we could raise children, and would enjoy doing so, and maybe, if we were lucky, they would come out of the experience relatively unscathed and definitely loved. Perhaps that is a bad, or a selfish, reason to want a family with someone, though I don't know what a good or a selfless reason is. But it's what I felt, what I still feel, and to deny it does no good.

Wouldn't it be easier if we could turn desire on and off? If we only wanted within reason?

There's a complex ethics of want, of course. Sometimes we want things that are bad for us, or for others, or both. Sometimes we want things we simply cannot have. Sometimes I want another beer even though I know I shouldn't, and the want weasels its way into my brain, and when I wake, heavy-headed and dry-mouthed, I wonder what possessed me.

Want possessed me. Want possesses all of us, for better or worse.

Now I think: I would like to be dispossessed of this particular want. I would like to take it or leave it, to be on the fence about it, to shrug about it, to be able to do as so many doctors and strangers and friends have advised, and stop thinking about it, so that it can happen of its own accord, or so that if it doesn't, I won't care, or at least I won't care as much. But I am gripped by the sense that it would be doing a disservice to my own sense of identity to deny it, and, more than that, that it would be impossible, at this point, to let it go. It took a decision in the mind to get here, to this place; it would take another to go back to the place before, and even then I'm not sure there is any way, really, of accessing the place before: it would have to be a new place, one which I'm not sure we're ready to contemplate yet.

No, there is nothing left to do but to acknowledge the want, to embrace it, even if this means risking failure. Even if it means miring ourselves here for longer, bedding ourselves in, holding ourselves up.

8

A Map of Here

What would it mean to name this place I'm in, to map it? To say: *this* is the landscape. It looks like this, smells like this, at night these are the sounds that carry on the wind. *Almost-motherhood.*

Well, you could try. The first thing to say is that there is no way to navigate here. There's no sea, no edge. The landscape is everywhere around you; you cannot move confidently in any direction and know where you might be headed. It is characterised by a kind of sameness, a repetition that both soothes and disorients. You might walk for miles and find yourself thinking: *but this looks just like where I was.* A desert, perhaps, a flat sky – even the horizon is obscured, or else it keeps moving further away.

Barren, a wasteland: but not entirely. There is life here, sometimes the sands shift, a tree shades the earth, a hill rises and falls, a bird or a bee catches your attention. But it is not a settled place. Because you never quite know where you are you are always on the back foot, late to appreciate the moments of beauty, afraid that in your disorientation you might languish here for too long, that you might be seduced to stay. The air engenders a kind of stupor, like being drugged: this is not the place to think sharply, to make quick decisions, to commit to anything but the one choice that landed you here. Sometimes a heavy fog descends, obscures the whole landscape. Sometimes it is clear as a mountain stream and the sun warms your back but something – a memory, perhaps, or a fear – clouds your senses all the same, makes you tense.

Or maybe it is simply this: a calm flat sea. The doldrums. The wind will not fill your sails. You are powerless here. Rescue will come, or it won't, but in the meantime all you can do is wait, and drift, and feel the world move around you.

9
Dolls

It is not quite true, of course, to say that I had never really thought about having children before I met Alexander. I have had a relationship with the idea of motherhood all my life. It is hard to be a woman and not to have had at some point this assumption foisted upon you: that your most basic ambition, indeed the entire purpose of your existence, your raison d'être, is to be a mother. Trace the assumption back far enough and you see that even in some of our earliest games we engage with it: the way we mother our dolls or our younger siblings, or role play with our own parents.

Do you want children? Or the presumptive version: *when are you going to have children?* If you are a woman of childbearing age – especially, although certainly not exclusively, if you are in a long-term, monogamous relationship with a man – you will know this question. At what point is it first asked of us, I wonder? When do we first learn that it is a question which, as women, we will need to find an answer for – even if that answer is not necessarily the one we ourselves hoped for, even if we do not want to answer, even if we do not yet have an answer?

The truth is that as a child I was particularly interested in pregnancy, in babies. I stuffed pillows under my shirt and waddled around in my bedroom, aping the awkward gait I had observed pregnant women adopting, the way they held their hands to their bellies. I asked my mother to call me 'Mommy';

she would play the child. Still an infant myself, I pretended a favourite doll was my own offspring, and looked tenderly after it, and was horrified when one day an arm fell off, whispered it to my parents with all the seriousness I could muster, as if it were a real crisis, and not one of imagination.

I don't know if this interest was because it was what I saw a lot of my parents' friends doing at the time – being pregnant, looking after babies and small children – or because I was an only child, and yearned in some almost imperceptible way for *another*, perhaps a smaller version of me, that I could mother, in a way. Perhaps it was because of my own relative proximity to the womb: a lingering body-memory, deeper than logic – *the security and irresponsibility* of that time before. Perhaps it was culturally inscribed, inescapable. But in a way thoughts of motherhood, although that's not how I would have described them, obsessed me from an early age.

I remember now a dream I had when I was about seven. In it, a version of me – not my actual seven-year-old body, but a *me* somehow outside time – was pregnant. A teacher at my elementary school, a small, middle-aged, grey-haired woman, approached me. How have *you* accomplished this while still so young, she asked in the dream, though not in those exact words, when I have spent my whole life trying to have a baby?

The dream made no sense to me then, makes no sense to me now; I did not even know, at that age, how pregnancy was achieved. But lately I have begun to fear that it was a kind of vision, or a premonition. The teacher wasn't the teacher (who, as far as I know, may well have had her own children in real life); the teacher was *me*, an older version of me.

Do I believe that? Of course not, and yet . . . and yet. Some little niggling doubt: what if my body, my subconscious, everything about me except my rational, waking, thinking mind, the mind writing these words, the mind that *wants*, knows something, understands something, about my own ability to reproduce? What if I am shouting at myself, into a void, into a seven-year-old's dream?

Or perhaps it means nothing, except to signify how deep-seated the desire is, how long this obsession has had to take root. If I want to trace its origins, I need to go back all the way to the role play, to the pillows, to the dolls. To the beginning. If I want to unpick it, understand it, I need to admit first of all how well woven it is into the fabric of my story, how completely – for better or for worse – I have internalised a narrative that is both intensely personal and also much bigger, much more expansive, than myself.

And then what? I won't want a baby any less just because I've overthought it, just because I've acknowledged the factors outside my control; want doesn't work like that. But better, perhaps, to admit the irrationality of it all than to try to fight it, to try to reason with it; better to float than to flail.

10

Us and Them

One day, over coffee, a friend mentions that her son has developed an interest in the first woman to swim the English Channel.

For a time after my friend gave birth to her son I used to go round to her house and help look after him so she could get some work done on a book whose deadline was approaching. Sometimes we would both sit at the kitchen table, the baby asleep in his Moses basket, trying to decipher difficult handwriting in a letter that might or might not be important. Sometimes if he was grizzly I would just carry him around the house while she worked, since movement seemed to be a soothing gesture. If there was music playing I would dance with him, turning in circles in the lounge. I didn't really know how to interact with babies, so often I chatted away to him as if he were an adult friend, as if he would be able to respond to my comments and questions with some sharp insight into the human condition.

When I saw this friend with her baby, even though she was older than me, even though she was married, with a house and a career and a nice handbag, it made me feel as if somehow it would be possible to be like that, to be both mother and myself, to be ambivalent about the particulars but also fluent in the physical and habitual language of parenthood. I guess until then I had not really thought about what it would mean to *be* a mother, only — and at this point in very cursory terms — to *become* one. Certainly I had not thought beyond the hazy, milky phase of birth and infancy, had not thought about the permanence of parenthood, the constant negotiation between mother-self and other-self, the grittiness of it, the actual *raising* of a child, into the teenage years and beyond: I had thought nothing of that.

My friend's son is a baby no longer. He is a fully fledged little human, with interests and ideas all his own. He loves swimming, and has identified as a particular heroine a woman called Gertrude Ederle, who he discovered in a book. I know the name, but little else about her, so we google her: she was American, an Olympian, a world record holder. She swam the Channel faster than any man ever had before, and her record stood for almost twenty-five years. But her career never really gained the momentum that this initial flurry of fame had promised, and she struggled financially as well as emotionally. In 1933 she fell down a set of stairs and gravely injured her back; she was told by doctors she might never walk or swim again, though in 1939 she was sufficiently recovered to perform in a water show at the New York World's Fair. Due to a childhood case of measles she had persistent hearing trouble, and by the 1940s she was almost completely deaf; for many years she taught deaf children to swim. She was agreeable to interviews about her Channel swim but hated to be pitied: *Don't weep for me, don't write any sob stories,* she reportedly told the *New York Times* in 1956. She never married, she never had children. She died in 2003, at the age of ninety-eight, at a nursing home in New Jersey, *survived by ten nephews and nieces.*

When I get home I look her up in Charles Sprawson's *Haunts of the Black Masseur,* in which I remember reading a reference to her, and I'm struck by his description of her defining feat:

When in 1926 Gertrude Ederle became the first woman to swim the Channel, swimming crawl all the way to beat the existing men's record by two hours, sirens greeted her on her return to New York, flowers showered down from planes, and the enthusiasm of her ticker-tape welcome equalled that of Lindbergh the following year. Unfortunately she lost millions in sponsorship when she delayed her return some months in order to visit a grandmother in Germany, and the Channel in the meantime was swum by a mother.

Reading this again, I get hung up on that last line. *The Channel in the meantime was swum by a mother* – a strange phrase: who was this mother, and why has she lost her right to be named? Why is her motherhood significant at all in this context? Why has the sentence been set up to imply that it makes her somehow an inferior athlete to Ederle, who was able presumably to devote her body and her mind more wholly to the endeavour? And why does Ederle's lack of motherhood also seem to be an implied weakness? That her feat could be replicated by a mere mother, well!

The 'mother' Sprawson refers to is Amelia 'Mille' Gade Corson, a Danish-American swimmer who had first attempted the Channel in 1923, nine months after giving birth to her first child. She finally made her successful crossing just three weeks after Ederle. In the preceding months, as the race to be the first woman to swim the Channel had heated up, her status as a mother had distinguished her from her rivals, especially for the press. In one article, headlined *MOTHER OF 2 WILL MAKE ANOTHER TRY TO SWIM CHANNEL*, she frames her motherhood as an asset: *I think no woman is at her best, physically or otherwise, until she is a mother,* she says. An offhand comment, perhaps, or one intended to offset the continual pressure to prove that one could be both a mother *and* anything else, the assumption of weakness read into her motherhood. And yet I find myself bridling, stung. *Her best, physically or otherwise.*

★

There's a certain kind of mum, a mumsy mum, that I have come to hate. There she is, in the pub, in the park, in the queue at the sandwich shop, rolling her pram patiently back and forth while she waits, glancing at her baby every few seconds, as if it might disappear, as if it might, in those gaps between glances, take on a life of its own, cease needing her so intensely, so viscerally. She wears clothing that doesn't fit her well anymore, too tight or too loose, or clothing clearly purchased for practicality. Her hair is in a ponytail, though wisps have escaped: a metaphor? She makes regular little public performances of Competent Motherhood. My least favourite is the ostentatious nappy-sniff. She lifts the baby out of the pram, or out of the arms of a friend or the father, and presses her nose to the white puff of its bottom. *Sniff, sniff*: audible from across a crowded room. If the baby has done a poo, which invariably it has, she will turn her head away suddenly, screw up her face. 'Whew!' she'll say, and then disappear, but not without making a fuss, without making extravagant motions to extract wipes and nappies from an overstuffed bag.

To her friends, who are also mumsy mums, she will describe notable bowel movements. She will bemoan the changes in her life, the lack of sleep, the lack of hours to get everything done. She will do this in a way that manages to make her seem simultaneously sad and smug.

I will sit at a table near them, and their conversation will drown out whatever I am thinking. What strikes me is not so much its banality – most conversation among friends is banal, how's work, how's family, the other day I had lunch at that Thai place you recommended, I'm thinking about buying a new toaster, and so on – but its insularity: the *we-ness* of it, which by necessity implies a *you*, an *other*. What I feel is that they see straight through me, by which I mean they do not see me sitting there at all, by which I mean that they see a woman of their own age and social standing without a baby, without a belly, and therefore without value, without utility. Without understanding of the complexity of their lives, by which I mean life in general.

What if they see this: nothing, no one, an empty chair – or worse, a waste of space?

If I could read the last four paragraphs back to myself and say, truthfully, that I had never thought that way, never felt that way, I would delete them. I would pretend they had never existed.

But what good is ugliness if all we do is keep it to ourselves? What good is pretending?

I remember that the first time I was pregnant, brief as it was, I felt an affinity, a reaching-out, towards other women who were pregnant – I wanted to draw them closer, to identify them, and for them to identify me, to form a kind of unspoken fellowship. Now you could say I feel the opposite, a revulsion, as if I repulse everyone, and everyone repulses me. The way I look at people, the way I look at the woman with her nose pressed to her baby's bottom, is mean, and deliberately so, and I know it, and maybe they know it too. I know I am creating my own distance, facilitating my own disappearance. I know I am the sole perpetrator. I know it isn't fair, or right.

But then I think about this: in her memoir *The Argonauts*, Maggie Nelson writes about what she calls a *hard season* in her relationship with her partner, and how, during this season, she sought some evidence that other seemingly happy couples had experienced unhappiness and persevered with their love anyhow. This search, she says, reminded her of what she describes as *a particularly dysfunctional moment* in the writer Leonard Michaels' fictionalised account of his volatile relationship with his first wife, Sylvia Bloch. In the scene Nelson is referring to, a friend describes to Michaels the horrible fights he has with his own wife. *It was an extraordinary moment*, Michaels writes. *I was grateful to him, relieved, giddy with pleasure. So others lived this way, too . . . Such thinking, like bloodletting, purged me. I was miserably normal; I was normally miserable.*

Nelson calls this moment dysfunctional, and I can see that, of course, not least because we know what happens next, in real life at least: that Bloch and Michaels are married sometime around 1960, and that she commits suicide in 1963; theirs is not a happy story. But I also see a kind of poignancy in it, something essentially human. I see myself in it. I think of the awful tingle of relief when, for example, I read an article about miscarriage or infertility that includes quotes from other women who have had experiences similar to mine; or when I learn that so-and-so doesn't have children, or couldn't; even when I meet someone who does, but who is open about how long it took, how difficult the process was. It's a complicated feeling: it sits alongside sadness, horror. It's terrible, yes, dysfunctional, to have these thoughts, and a part of me, as I'm having them, is acutely aware that I don't want anybody to be unhappy, to suffer misfortune, to experience sadness or pain. But at the same time the knowledge that others have, others do, eases my own discomfort.

So others lived this way, too: I don't want to be alone. I don't want to disappear. No, rephrase that: it's a fear, not a desire. I'm afraid of being alone. Afraid of disappearing.

★

Why am I so fixated on all this – *the Channel in the meantime was swum by a mother*? Why am I so sensitive to the language, the word *mother*, so intent on reading something into it, treating it like an affront? Why does it make me defensive, when I have nothing to defend?

The answer is obvious: envy. Thwarted desire. Uncertainty. Self-preservation. The real question, the more interesting question, is this: what if we disappear no matter what? If we become mothers, if we don't. If we're somewhere in between, if there isn't a name for the place we are except *here*, if choice, want, desire has been taken away from us, or foisted upon us, or questioned, or doubted, or twisted for someone else's purposes.

Us and them, and a canyon in between: but the neatness of this, like so many neatnesses, is false. What if we spoke across the divide, as if motherhood and non-motherhood were not binary but complementary states, as if we were not handmaids and wives but simply women, with messy, leaky, miraculous, disobedient bodies? As the new mother feels alone, the non-mother, the almost-mother, the once-mother, the would-be mother, feels alone; there is nothing to say that one experience can't speak to the other, even that we can't be alone together.

The truth is this: that I do hate them, those women in the pub, in the park, in the queue at the sandwich shop, those mumsy mums. Not all the time, but sometimes, yes. That I hate them because I am afraid of becoming them, and also, more pressingly, because I am afraid of not becoming them. I have flattened them, oversimplified them for my own personal appeasement: too difficult to acknowledge their own internal complexities, the things they've abandoned unwillingly, the possibility – the likelihood – that what they see in the mirror is not what I see from across the café, is not what they expected to see, or wanted to see, or like to see. It is sometimes too much of a stretch of imagination, too great an act of empathy on an angry stomach, to see the universality of the fear, of the loneliness, to see how the way they position their prams is done with both care and external anxiety, that they don't want to inconvenience people, or get in the way, or that they have ceased caring because something else more pressing is weighing on them, or that when the baby is finally asleep a great relief, for a moment, washes over them. Too hard, when you're tired, when you're afraid, even to look across the canyon, let alone speak across it.

But try.

So much of this, in the end, is to do with want, and with what women want in particular. What if a woman doesn't want a baby, but has one growing anyhow? What if she does want one, but things – time, financial or cultural pressures, her own body – conspire against it? Why are we so afraid of both scenarios, so afraid to let want be want – as if it might cause the fabric of society to fray, to not interrogate a want, to not challenge it, to not try to read deeper meaning into it, to not demand justification or payment for it, or in any case to regulate it?

Besides, there often is no clear-cut decision: the world is not neatly divided into two camps of women, those who wanted to reproduce and did, and those who didn't want to, and didn't. So many of us are caught here, in between, neither one thing nor the other, drifting towards a receding horizon, in our own camp. It could still go one way or the other for us: for the women who have not yet conceived in spite of years of trying, for the women who have lost pregnancies for no identifiable reason – or indeed for an identifiable one; for the women who have frozen their eggs, for the women who are seeking a partner, or whose partners might have different wants, one way or the other. For the women who have decided one thing but may in time, quite simply, change their minds.

Even among those for whom there has been an 'outcome', an ending of sorts to the story, a beginning to a new one, there's a fuzziness to it all. Many of the women I know who do not have children, biological or otherwise, did not actively choose not to – indeed some of them chose the opposite, and then found it impossible, or else they never found a partner with whom they wanted to have, or raise, a child, or else they simply waited on the decision, until it made itself. Meanwhile, it's equally possible, equally likely, to feel ambivalent about motherhood but find yourself, or make yourself, a mother anyhow – or even for that choice to have been foisted on you, or taken away from you, or made for you.

There's something, too, about wanting and complaining: a cult of silence around what happens after you *get what you want*. Women who yearn for a pregnancy, for example, are expected to keep mum about their discomfort once it's achieved, *because it was wanted*. Ditto a marriage, a family, a life, everything: if you wanted it, you can't complain. But want is not absolute. You can want something knowing it will not bring you all the happiness in the world, knowing that it will make things more complicated, less comfortable. You can want something and then get it and be grateful to have it and still hold in your head the idea that it isn't exactly as you expected, or hasn't filled all the holes in your life, or is in its own way much more challenging than not having it. You can look across the fence at the neighbours' garden, differently arranged, and envy them, even when you wouldn't change anything, not really, and can't anyway.

If I know this, can I also then start to imagine a scenario whereby it is possible to *not* get what I want, or for the route to be different than I imagined it would be, longer and harder, and to not feel resentful? Can I start to imagine a scenario whereby my own pain, such as it is, is a smooth part of my body, that it does not work against me, that it does not insist on pitting me against others?

Not yet, no, not yet.

But someday?

Someday, yes.

11

Weight

Somewhere along the way the ripe spring, overripe now, has tipped into the lime-green tangy promise of early summer. A friend is getting married in September, and she asks if I'd like to go to an exercise class with her on Monday evenings. She wants to lose some weight, she says, not a lot, but a little, so that when she puts on the thin silk gown she has picked out for the wedding she will feel her best. I know that feeling, the feeling that somehow to look my best, to be my best, requires me to make parts of myself disappear, although perhaps that isn't exactly what she means.

Why is being a woman, I think, so often about growing and shrinking, shrinking and growing?

The class is run by an enthusiastic redhead who blasts a Beyoncé-heavy soundtrack through her laptop and coaxes us into increasingly frenzied synchronised movement, half dance, half old-school aerobics. My friend and I position ourselves at the back, where the neat rows of women who have been coming for weeks and who know the routine can't see how sloppy we are, how we go left when the instructor yells right, how when she asks us to hold our arms out to the side and pulse them for minutes on end we give up early, or how sometimes, unsure of how to execute a particular movement, we simply stand there and laugh.

After the first class I am so sore for the rest of the week that I can barely walk up the stairs to bed. Well, good, I find myself thinking: perhaps I need this, or deserve it. Not quite penance, but something like it. To make my body *do* something. To make it hurt, at least a little, in aid of strength, resilience. Or at least not to waste its vital youth sitting around in the evenings doing nothing.

But, too, I find myself again trying to hold multiple possibilities in my body at once. Alexander and I return to the fertility clinic, where they write me another prescription for clomifene; I fill it. On Monday evenings I start to wonder abstractly: is this kind of exercise bad if you're trying to conceive? If you might – probably aren't but *might*, because it is technically possible – be pregnant?

And then there are moments that I enjoy it, or that I feel at least that there is still the potential for pleasure even in a state of more general ambiguity. My friend and I walk part of the way home together, past the coffee roastery, the Samaritans, the Buddhist centre, the church. We part at the corner shop with the vegetables in crates outside, under hot grey evening skies, the whole rest of the week stretching in front of us, the rest of the summer, really, and my muscles feel tired, and heavy in a good way, like I have some weight to me, some substance.

I am still angry. There's no getting around it. Will I ever not be angry? Even if everything, eventually, goes our way – will there ever be a time when I do not feel as if something, somehow – an innocence, if nothing else, the prospect of a pregnancy without the weight of constant anxiety – has been taken from me?

But what I've begun to see is that it's possible to feel, to be, two things at once. I can be angry, and yet still experience pleasure; I can be angry and still feel fundamentally OK, day to day, month to month: the anger needn't erupt, I can keep it more or less in check, so that it only bubbles up occasionally, when I am tired or drunk or stressed. I can worry about what might or might not come, but at the same time I can also hold a sense of the future as full, as promising: just because you don't know what it is doesn't mean that it won't be something good.

Do I really believe that? Perhaps I do.

Five

An Inscription

2016–2017

I

Begin Again

I have got back into the swing of swimming. I have started to run again, a little. On Monday evenings I go to the aerobics class with my friend, and we chat on the way there, the way home. Isn't a life just built out of routines, repetitions? Annie Dillard's *How we spend our days is, of course, how we spend our lives*: which is to say that while I have been stuck, drifting on the windless sea, while I have been waiting for the elusive *until*, my life has been taking shape. Or perhaps more accurately, it has always had shape; there is no such thing as a shapeless life; I may still feel invisible sometimes, watching those mumsy mums, but I have not in fact disappeared, have not dissolved.

Early in the summer my boss at the office takes me out to lunch, a cafeteria-style restaurant in the centre of town that smells of over-warmed lasagne. We sit across from each other at a table by the window. My contract with the company is up in a few months, in September. We have already renewed it once, late last year, on mutual agreement. We have talked a little, since, about my role, about how we might expand or tailor it to my interests and skills, in a way that implies I might have a future there, if I want it, even though I think in many ways I have done a very bad job, I have hardly cared at all about the company, its strategic aims, its profit margins or lack thereof. During these conversations I have often been noncommittal, vague, because I am not sure what I want. I took the job initially because it was fixed-term, part-time, afforded me some financial security while I saw through the final year of my PhD. I was grateful for it, but I remember too that the day I signed the contract, I came home and burst into tears. All afternoon, all evening, I couldn't stop crying, I felt as if I had done something wrong, as if I had made some great mistake. Alexander held me very close when he came home but I couldn't explain the tears: was it to do with having made a commitment, even a short-term one, to something when everything else – by which I mean the question of whether we would or would not be able to have a baby – was still up in the air? Or maybe it was just the sulkiness of the July heat, a delayed post-wedding comedown, the awkward negotiation I'd had about my salary, I don't know. But when, talking it through with Alexander, I tried to identify what it was exactly that made me so uncomfortable, the only tangible thing I could put my finger on was that the hours would mean I couldn't go to the pool at my usual time anymore, that I'd have to get there earlier, and this made it seem, more than anything else, as if my entire world were shifting, slipping away from me: how would I know who I was any more, where I stood, if I could not continue to do my laps at exactly the same time each morning?

But now sometimes in the toilets at the office, washing my hands, I will glance up at the mirror and think: do I want what this *could* be, the promise of security, the full-time nine-to-five, the chair with lumbar support, the two screens, the responsibility of watering the office plants, the occasional drinks with co-workers, the share options, the Friday relief, the Sunday anxiety? And I have to admit that in some ways this is not unappealing. It is simple, understandable. If I have a baby, I think, I would have paid maternity leave, and a job to come back to, a stable income with which, in combination with Alexander's salary, we could perhaps get a mortgage, a house, or at least a flat, it would be the responsible thing to do.

Have I given any thought, my boss asks now, to what I would like to do in September, when my contract is up?

I tell him: I need to finish my PhD thesis, once and for all. I don't think, realistically, I can do that and renew my contract. I'm sorry.

The relief on both sides of the table is palpable.

I don't know what this means for anything else, this decision, but it feels good, at least, to make a choice, and to feel that I have some ownership of my future, my time. On my lunch breaks, when it's sunny, I go and sit in the shade of a tree in a nearby park and make plans. I print out a calendar and mark out various PhD deadlines; I begin to seek freelance work; I think about what now, what next. Perhaps it is after all possible to move forward without relinquishing hope and desire for the thing we want but cannot control: perhaps the landscape of almost, of maybe, can accommodate some growth.

I also have the clomifene. This in itself is a hopeful thing. It worked before, I think. Surely it will work again. I don't think about beyond that, about what I would feel if it did, about the shadow the two miscarriages would cast. I cannot, or it would be impossible to take any action at all; I would be well and truly stuck in place, rooted by fear.

*

I remember, years ago, just after my first miscarriage, talking to a friend, who was pregnant with her second child at the time, about the worry of a miscarriage, the mistrust it engenders. I wonder, I'd said, if I get pregnant again, if I'll ever be able to relax. And she said she understood, but that really that sense of worry never left you, it just evolved. Even once you had a baby – *especially* once you had a baby – you were always a little on edge, always standing on the brink of the terrifying unknown. There's always something else to worry about, she'd said, which was strangely a comfort: to know that in a way we are all here, suspended between hope and fear, in a state of perpetual unknowing, even those of us who seem to have it all, who seem to have transitioned into parenthood so effortlessly. To know that other people must and do find ways of coping with the ache of uncertainty, that it is in a sense the most basic human condition there is, something we all share, whoever and wherever we are, made me feel less alone, even in a moment when I had cause to feel alone, a moment when I might even have found the comment hurtful.

In truth I had long been jealous of these particular friends, though I would not have necessarily phrased it that way. It had become a point of pain between Alexander and I: whenever my bitterness about how their situation measured up to ours – about what exactly, their lovely life, their house with its shiny new kitchen, their apparent ease in the world? – became palpable, he would try to shut it down. I can't have this conversation with you, he would say, teeth on edge. Fine, I would snap back, unable to see it from his point of view, the way I was managing to be cruel both to us and to our friends.

I remember in particular the way I felt when they announced that they were expecting their first baby – I was at their house on a cold, dark, winter afternoon, sipping tea, and they produced a little photo, an image from a scan. She had been weak and ill with the symptoms of early pregnancy but was now starting to emerge out the other side, into the relative vitality of the second trimester. I was happy for them but also somehow shocked; I felt immediately and illogically as if I were being left behind, as if in telling me their good news they were also telling me that our friendship was over. I don't know why I felt this so keenly: this was over a year before Alexander and I made our own decision to have a baby; I was still on birth control, still ostensibly unready to be a mother myself, did not feel jealous of their *pregnancy* so much, I suppose, as I did of their unborn baby, who would get so much of the attention that I felt was somehow owed to the other people in their lives who had been there first. Petty, selfish, yes, but it was an instinctual reaction, not one I could control or even articulate, not for years after. I was just about able to feel myself drawing away from them in response to the news, and Alexander, who seemed able to be unreservedly happy for them, to separate himself entirely from the situation, bridled at my barely disguised spite.

Their son was born that July, and the day we went to meet him for the first time was summer-clear and mild. We sat outside on the terrace in their back garden, in wicker chairs with padded seats. We drank tea and passed the baby around. He was tiny, mostly asleep, sweet and beautiful in the way that your friends' babies always are. His parents looked tired and stunned and happy all at once. We stayed for an hour or two and then caught a bus back towards town. We got off at the train station, but the evening was young and warm and light, so rather than changing to the bus for home we walked to a bar nearby. We ordered pints of cold lager in sweating glasses and carried them to the outside seating area, an alleyway squeezed between the bar and a scuzzy nightclub. The sun hit our faces before it dipped behind the club. We talked about – what, exactly? All kinds of things. The weather, the season, our friends, their baby. We ordered another pint, and then another. It was easy and pleasant to be there, to sit and chat, to be happy for our friends and also happy for ourselves and the luxury of that long, meandering summer's day, even though if I'm honest our relationship had not necessarily been easy and pleasant of late.

We'd been through a rough patch. No: let's call it a period of restlessness. I in particular had no sense of direction, no purpose, nothing to galvanise me in the mornings or excite me in moments of private contemplation, and this listless despera-tion seeped into our relationship. I began to feel that we were somehow growing distant from each other, that perhaps we had outgrown whatever it was we had once had, or not grown enough. We never had any money: this was a strain, perhaps *the* strain, though we didn't quite see it at the time. The previous year I had left a good but dull job as an account manager for a web development agency but was not now bringing in enough as a freelance writer to justify the decision; he, meanwhile, had recently abandoned a comparatively lucrative freelance career to work at a start-up that couldn't really afford to pay him yet. Sometimes I woke up in the mornings and thought: *this isn't working*, but I didn't know exactly what 'this' was. Me? Us? I fantasised about leaving – not him, exactly, but this situation, our life as it was. We could go elsewhere, do other things, except that we couldn't, we were somehow tied to where we were, the only way to get out of the slump was to stay and fight.

I had, meanwhile, secretly applied for a PhD programme. Without telling Alexander, or anyone, I took a train to Egham one blustery March afternoon to meet with a potential supervisor. Waiting on the platform after I remember thinking: *if I'm accepted, I promise I'll pour all my energy into this, I'll get as much out of it as I possibly can.* Of course that wouldn't be exactly how things panned out, of course I had unrealistic expectations about what the PhD would actually mean, but when I was accepted it gave me some equilibrium back; it gave me something to focus on, something to aim for. Something to tell people at parties. It made even our relationship seem fresh again: this idea that I had some value, some purpose, even if the actual nature of that purpose was ambiguous, eased the strain, allowed me to see, or start to see, the good in us again.

And I remember this: that evening, after visiting our friends and their new baby, as the sky was fading and the shadows lengthening, Alexander looked at me and said, you know, we should be . . . *nicer* to each other.

I knew instinctively what he meant, and when he said it, it sounded simple. It is not so simple to enact, of course, but actually, as it turns out, it is not so hard, either. A kind of reset button, beginning again, except with deeper knowledge of each other, a more entwined history, a more realistic set of expectations about what it means to live with someone and build a life together. Be nicer to each other: why had we forgotten to do this? What had made us remember? Perhaps it was watching our friends and their baby – a family – folding in on each other, enclosing each other, becoming a unit, and understanding that at the end of the day we too came home to no one but each other, that we were a unit too, in our own way. Perhaps it was just the pleasantness of the moment, the bar, the beer, the faded sky, the last of the sunlight.

When you love someone, and they love you, it is easy, too easy, to forget to engage with that love, to work and adapt. When Alexander and I first met I remember looking at other couples – strangers, friends – and thinking: *what they have is nothing compared to what we have.* I remember thinking that their love was – not inferior, exactly, but simply not comparable. The power, the purity, of our love, was unlike anything that anyone else had. I did not know that of course this is a thing that many people think at the start of an intense relationship, especially when you are both very young. But for a long time after that – too long; years! – I had relied purely on the strength of those feelings, the love, the hate, the kissing, the shouting, to sustain us. I had assumed that they would, that they could. When really nothing can sustain you but yourselves, and all the banal work you do, all the little moments, the bus rides and the beers, the conscious decisions to keep going, to be kind.

*

The month I'm meant to restart the clomifene we go to Wales for a long weekend. My period is due a few days before we leave, and when it still hasn't come on the day of our departure I wonder, though at first only abstractly. It's a hot day, sunny, blue sky and puffy clouds. A Friday afternoon: we are stuck on the A40 in bank holiday traffic, our car has no air conditioning, we roll the windows down and turn the radio up. I cast my mind back – how did I feel with my other pregnancies at this stage, are there any signs, is there anything I can grab on to? I identify a vague nausea – car sickness, probably, the heat, but what if . . . ? Somewhere along the way we stop for petrol and

I unroll a sweet, a Werther's Original, partially melted, and while Alexander pays for the petrol the thought that has been forming solidifies at last: I should take a test. I'll buy one over the weekend, I think. Something warm seems to settle in my chest, in my belly. A secret, a hope, a palpable presence.

How is it possible that even now, even after all these years, I can still feel like this, can still play this game? The next evening, at dinner, I think: tomorrow, if my period still hasn't come, I'll go into the pharmacy in town. But in the middle of the night I wake to a pain, and a full bladder, and when I go to the bathroom I see that it was all in my imagination, this presence, this neat little story, and so the next morning, as instructed, with a sigh, I take the clomifene, begin again.

2

Out of Place

We've always been good at talking, Alexander and I. We've talked and talked, backwards and forwards, about anything and everything. It's what we do, what we've always done, what everything is built on: that night we met, the way we talked for hours and hours and hours, and all the nights after. A favourite weekend indulgence has always been to find a pub on a sunny afternoon and to stay there all evening, talking our way through the world. Current events, major life decisions, childhood recollections dredged up out of nowhere, things we've read recently, things we've seen recently. Politics, ethics, art, farts, the whole shebang.

We have talked, of course, about where we are, at least obliquely, about this long ongoing moment, the difficulty of Our Current Situation. But it is harder and harder to find a language for it, a way of communicating what we each actually feel in a way that is both empathetic and honest. And for some time now it has felt as if we have exhausted all possible conversations on the subject of pregnancy, or lack thereof. We still talk, but only in circles. I have been angry and he has been conciliatory; he has been angry and I have been conciliatory. I have said unkind things about us both and he has listened and then gone outside and drawn on a cigarette and forgiven me, again. He has held his tongue when perhaps *he* would like for once to say the unkind things, but even so he has sometimes done unkind things, I think without realising, or without meaning to: coming home late, drunk, when I have been texting, when he has said he is on his way but not meant it; not taking my side when I have felt stung or slighted by someone else's actions, justly or unjustly. I don't even know what I would like to get out of the conversations that so often turn into fights. Perhaps these days it would be better simply not to say anything, not to speculate: the subject is too fraught, we become unlike ourselves the deeper we wade in, as if we have forgotten that we in fact are on the same side. *Be nicer to each other.* But I cannot seem to help myself.

For example: one evening, struggling to sleep, I sit up straight in bed, full of fury. I have recently had my period again, started the next round of clomifene, begun again, again. 'I'm never fucking pregnant,' I say. I want to talk about the unfairness of it all, or rather, I want to *complain* about the unfairness of it all, I want to say both that I am useless and also that it isn't my fault. I speak in circles. What did I do to deserve this? Nothing! But also obviously I'm inferior somehow, obviously I'm incapable, obviously I *do* deserve it. But also isn't it unfair? Isn't it unjust? He talks to me for a while, but it's impossible. All I want is to be angry, not to be soothed or talked round. He gets up, goes downstairs; I smell the smoke drifting up through the open window, an old habit that rears its head in times of stress or anxiety.

It's always a test, these days: of faith, of loyalty, of the strength of our relationship, of patience.

How long have we been like this? How long has it been since sex wasn't scheduled, since it didn't feel like a *waste* if it wasn't on a potentially fertile day – the mutter that tonight would be a good night, the ovulation stick has indicated a luteinising hormone surge – since we talked, at the end of an evening, of anything other than fertility? I lie there breathing hard while he is outside, thinking that this is no way to be in a relationship, it's no good for either of us, it's not who we are. I know it isn't; I know we are each, in our own way, aching on behalf of the other; I know if I would only soften, apologise, then things would be easier, everything would feel better even if no funda-mental problem had been solved, we could lie as we usually do, folded close together, the weight of each other's limbs a balm. I have learned some things over the years. But when he comes back upstairs, to bed, I roll deliberately away, facing the wall, my eyes shut as if in sleep.

Later that week I start to bleed, mid-cycle. I am late for work at the office, and I think little of it at the time; my brain is slow to register the strangeness of it, the unlikeliness. I think, *it must be the clomifene, a side effect.* But it is not listed among the numerous side effects in the information leaflet, and later that day, sitting at my desk, staring out at the rooftops, I feel a strange pain deep down that makes me sit up straight and think urgently, *something's wrong.* I phone a doctor at the clinic who have prescribed the clomifene. He asks me a few questions and then suggests that in spite of my conviction that, for once, I can't possibly be pregnant, I take a test.

Positive.

This is not happy news. Right off the bat, something is wrong; for a start it means that my last period was not in fact a period, that I have in fact been bleeding inexplicably, on and off, for two weeks. Even so, is there a moment, even a tiny fraction of a moment, after I look at the test and see the two lines – but faint! – and feel that rush, the world shifting, the possibility? Yes, of course. Of course there is. I call Alexander into the bath-room and we examine the test together: yes, definitely positive, even though that second line is not very strong. Undeniable. We smile at each other; we can't help it. And then, quickly, we become pragmatic: what does this mean? We can't know for sure, we agree, so there's no point in panicking, but certainly it does not feel like the other positive tests, the wild, guarded optimism of them.

I phone the doctor back and I can hear an edge of concern, of interest, in his voice, but like the lines on the test it's faint.

Am I in any pain? he asks. I have to admit that no, I am not, not really, not at this moment, although I have had some pain, discomfort really. He arranges a scan in a few weeks. In the meantime it's a wait-and-see situation, as they so often are: call if anything changes, but otherwise proceed as normal. So all that week I keep going to work, I keep working on my PhD thesis, I keep doing things like having dinner with friends, going to the dentist, folding the laundry. We have new neighbours, a Danish couple and their two children, and one evening after dinner they invite us over for a drink. We sit outside on the patio and I sip my glass of red very slowly, unsure about whether I should be drinking at all. Whatever is going on, I reason, one glass won't make any difference. We sit there until past midnight; I decline the Japanese whisky, though I would like nothing more in the moment than to surrender myself to the sting of it, to stumble drunkenly back over the garden fence at the end of the night, as Alexander does. Instead I am stone cold sober when we go to bed, wired, my teeth clenched in spite of the pleasantness of the evening, the gentle pleasure of learning that next door to you, so close you can hear the children singing after school through the thin shared walls, are people that you genuinely like.

All the while – at dinner, at the dentist, folding the laundry, getting to know the neighbours – I am bleeding, lightly but definitively, held in a state of ignorant suspense. Another contour line in the terrain of almost, of maybe: I am pregnant, but perhaps not really, not in the sense that other women are, *normal women*, I think; the shadow of doubt was cast even before the two lines appeared on the test, and now I have to imagine somehow multiple possibilities at once, and know that only one can be true, and carry on anyway.

The thing, the wall, the hard fact that I keep coming up against, is this: nothing can be done, nothing can be known, *yet*. It takes time for an understanding of what's happening to be reached because of the fragility, the not-knowing, that characterises so much of any kind of early pregnancy, even a healthy one. *Pregnancy begins as speculation*, writes Joanne O'Leary, pointing out that for most of history there was no definitive way for medical professionals, let alone women themselves, to confirm a pregnancy until it had begun to show, or until a woman felt the 'quickening', the first movement of the foetus in the womb. The hormone detected by modern pregnancy tests, human chorionic gonadotropin (hCG), was only discovered in 1927, and even then there was still a long way to go before those little boxes of plastic sticks would appear in the 'Family Planning' aisle of Boots.

But still, even now, even when it's possible to pee on a stick and know within three minutes if you're pregnant or not, there's an awful lot of unknowing, of speculation, of reliance upon invisible indicators within the body itself in the early days and weeks of a pregnancy. Subtle changes or clues might, but might not, give you the answer you seek – and anyway, as O'Leary also points out, *bodies can be unreliable narrators*. Doctors are wary of being equivocal about anything at this stage except the fact that they can't be certain until they are, and although it has not been my experience, it's true that sometimes things really can be fine even if they look otherwise. So I limit the extent of my projections. I think only about this hour, this day, the end of the week maybe, at a stretch. I think about what I will wear to the wedding we're due to attend in a few weeks, the bride is seven months pregnant, what will make *me* look enviable? At the same time, I try to assume nothing, try to put myself in suspended animation: another kind of double life.

Until the doctors have a clearer picture of what is going on, swimming is inadvisable. Just as well; as much as I want the reassurance of regularity, I don't want to bring this unruly, unwanted possibility there, to the place of repetition and routine, the place where predictability rules, the clean place. Instead I walk, circling the neighbourhood. I frequent the parks on our side of town, pausing sometimes to look out towards the city's spires, pressed against the summer sky, or at the blue-brown skin of the river, where in the evening rowers glide along, dipping their oars at rhythmic intervals.

As I walk I tell myself various stories, though the only ones I want to repeat are the hopeful ones: that maybe I've imagined the whole thing; that everything is fine; that even if it isn't, it will be.

One of my colleagues at the office has recently announced that his wife is expecting their second baby. One day, mid-morning, mid-meeting, he takes a phone call. He steps out of the office to take it and when he comes back in he is visibly shaken. His wife, the baby, he's sure everything is fine but . . .

Everyone says: go, go! Another male colleague, who has a two-year-old child, who is very good at what he does but often quite spiky in social interactions, is especially understanding. You don't want to mess around with these things, he says. He says it knowingly.

I want to say something knowingly too. I want to make my colleague understand somehow that while all this is going on, here is another woman who is bleeding, who is scared, who knows what that particular fear tastes like. But I cannot think of anything knowing or comforting or even banal to say. I cannot speak at all. I cannot even move. I sit rooted to my chair. I wheel it back to my desk after the meeting and stare at my screen, answering emails with a kind of mechanical sharpness. When my colleague comes back two hours later – relaxed, relieved, everything's fine – still I feel rooted to the spot, invisible and exposed at the same time, dripping with my own dread, my own fear. I have nothing spare for my colleague, for his wife, not now, not at this particular moment. It is my own failing, but it is also unavoidable.

The thing the doctor is worried about, that I am worried about, is that my symptoms match those of an ectopic pregnancy:

literally a pregnancy *out of place*, where the egg has implanted itself outside the womb, usually in a fallopian tube. Rare, but not so rare: a one in ninety chance, maybe.[3] Potentially life threatening, since the tube is liable to rupture if the pregnancy goes untreated. (*Untreated!* I think: like an illness, an infection. The thing I want is souring in my body.) There is no situation, with an ectopic pregnancy, in which the embryo can be saved, and so I am suddenly defensive, wanting to protect my own body against this strange intruder, yearning only for the most ordinary physical sensations: the end of a run, not even a hard run, just an ordinary one, when your chest burns slightly and then you can stop; the sun on your back in a pub garden, the chill of a bottle of beer fresh from the fridge, the warmth it spreads.

Somewhere I read a reference to people 'battling infertility'. I think: to go to battle, one has to have an enemy. Is the enemy my own body? I have bridled against this idea in the past but now I think, *in this case, yes*, unequivocally and impossibly yes, and I want instinctively to protect it from itself. I yearn above all for routine: for the solidity and simplicity of my morning swim, the nods of the other women, the trace of chlorine on my hands later. Without this I seem to know nothing: not my own body, certainly, a perpetual mystery; not this city, which has taken on a different colour now that something so fundamental is so uncertain; not my own purpose, even on a minute scale. *What was it again?* I find myself asking, trying to identify the word I want, trying to remember why I opened a tab in my browser, trying to collect my thoughts.

What was it again? What was it? Where is it now? No answer occurs to me: everything feels too slippery, entirely ungraspable, or like a long rope is being rapidly unbraided.

3

The In-Between Room

For ten days I sit tight, or try to. I hold on to the comfort of the everyday, little anchoring things: the bins are collected on Thursday mornings, pulling me from sleep early; the postman, who has been delivering our post for almost a decade now, waves hello if he can see me through the glass of the front door; in the evenings I can hear through the walls the new neighbours' small son crying, protesting the necessity of a bath or railing against the unfairness of bedtime. At night I watch episode after episode of *Game of Thrones*, where shock and sex and violence are the only currencies, and during the day I try to work, to walk, to believe my own stories. I could almost keep going like this.

Almost. Eventually, inevitably, the roar of my own panic gets so loud that I can't hear anything else. I call my GP surgery on a Friday, get an emergency appointment late that afternoon. I am seen by a doctor I've never met before, a woman with a crisp, soothing voice. She has a medical student in with her and with my permission, as she examines me, she narrates to him what she is doing. 'See, the test is positive,' she says, indicating the vial of my pee on her desk. She asks if I am in pain right now. I consider. On the whole I have to say no, not really. I can feel nothing at all except the thrum of my own heart. She asks how long it has been since my last period, a difficult question to answer, as it turns out. She asks if I've been feeling ill, or dizzy. Then she asks me to go back out to the waiting room for a few minutes, if I don't mind.

I don't mind. While I sit I take my phone out of my pocket, scroll through Twitter. Sitting there I feel a sharpness, a stabbing deep within, and I regret not saying *yes, actually, I am still in pain*, even though it's intermittent, even though it comes and then when it goes I remember it only as a trace of what it was, faint again like the lines on the test, a ghost of itself. Why can I never say things like that, even when the doctor is asking, even when she is giving me every opportunity? Why do I want to somehow mitigate the impact of my own words, my own symptoms, my own physicality, my own existence?

It's because I can't help but question the validity of my physical experience: *this pain, is it enough, really, to warrant the word?* Because I think, too, that if I am quiet and meek and obedient then so will be my body; because I think that perhaps, after everything, I have lost the right to be certain about anything when it comes to my reproductive organs. What do I know? Nothing. I keep scrolling and the pain fades, but the uneasiness sits heavy still.

After a while, ten minutes maybe, the GP brings me back into the examination room. The medical student stands in a corner and I take a seat by the desk. It is nearly six o'clock, the surgery seemingly empty except for the three of us in this room. The GP's demeanour is so calm that I do not pick up on the signs of urgency until later. The thing we worry about with these symptoms, she says, is ectopic pregnancy. Yes, I say; that's what I'm worried about too. I'm sure that's not what's going on, she says, but just in case, *just in case*, I'm going to book you an appointment at the urgent gynaecology clinic this evening. Then she asks, offhandedly, how I got to the surgery. I tell her I walked, as if to prove that I am fine – could I have walked all the way from my house if something was really wrong, if I was really in any danger? If something really was wrong, could I have marched across the bridge in my flipflops and my sunglasses, passing slower pedestrians, enjoying the feeling of the sun on my back, the wink of the river below?

I know I could, of course, and she knows I could, and she says, well, look, I'm just going to book you a taxi. Just to save you the hassle of trying to get yourself to the hospital at rush hour, on a bus, or . . .

She makes it sound like nothing. The taxi picks me up outside the surgery. On the way to the hospital I text Alexander, who's at work in London, who doesn't know that I've taken myself to see the GP. *Leaving now,* he texts back immediately, but still it will be hours until he's here, with the Friday evening traffic. I feel suddenly embarrassed – about pulling him away, about being in a taxi when I would have been perfectly capable of getting a bus. To try to fool the taxi driver – but really myself – into thinking that I am not a *patient,* I tell him entirely unnecessarily that I'm visiting someone, and ask him to drop me off at the main hospital entrance. I pay my fare and wait for him to drive off before I walk away, towards the Women's Centre.

The urgent gynaecology clinic is grim and functional, peopled by deeply empathetic and capable staff, but lacking in any external warmth or hospitality. It's a mess, a maze, a windowless rabbit warren of corridors and locked doors and small strange rooms that no one wants to be in. It is attached to the maternity ward but accessed during the day via a side entrance, as if to separate the faulty women from the functional ones. Because I'm arriving after hours, I have to use the main entrance. I find myself holding the door for an enormously pregnant woman, her companion burdened by several visibly heavy bags, on her way, perhaps, to deliver her baby. He pauses as they pass a vending machine and she says to him with some impatience, 'not now!' She looks relieved when I decline to join them in the lift – they're heading up, I'm heading down.

At the clinic, I sit for a few hours in one of those small strange rooms that no one wants to be in, reading. It's a good book, which is a shame, since I'm hardly able to appreciate it. I read the same page a dozen times or more, maybe, and marvel at the fact that I can understand each individual word, that I can move my gaze across the page, and yet have no sense of how the words fit together, of what is being said. I find myself gazing up at regular intervals, narrating my situation in the voice of the author of the book. There isn't much to narrate, to be honest; nothing happens, for a long time no one comes to see me except very occasionally, to reassure me that the doctor will be here soon, but what is soon, a minute or an hour or an evening? The room is an examination room. The centrepiece is a gurney. Above the gurney is a poster explaining how to give CPR to adults and to children. There are dozens of printouts taped to walls and drawers, labels, instructions, notices. The door is kept closed, and the lights flicker, and I have no phone signal, which is frankly a relief. I log on to the hospital Wi-Fi to let Alexander know where I am, then log off and put my phone in my pocket, so I can't be tempted to google my symptoms yet again.

I'm seen by a succession of nurses and doctors, escalating in seniority as the evening wears on. They do what they can: a blood test, a few cursory checks, pressing my abdomen with cold, practised hands, asking me repeatedly if I feel 'well in myself', a difficult question to answer with any conviction, since anxiety has made me feel, maybe, things that aren't there, just as it's made me minimise the things that are, the ghost pain, the fear. They say reassuring things but ask me to come in over the weekend for another blood test, so that they can monitor my levels of hCG, the pregnancy hormone; in a normal pregnancy levels should increase steadily during the early weeks, whereas with an ectopic pregnancy levels may rise at a much slower rate, or stagnate completely. I already have a scan scheduled on Tuesday, and they are keen not to do one before unless absolutely necessary – the longer we can wait to do it, they say, the more conclusive it will be.

At this point it is fairly clear to me – and no doubt to them – what is going on. With mounting unease I recall the GP's soothing voice, her calm assuredness: she acted this way, I see now, not because she didn't believe that something is wrong with me but precisely because she *did*, precisely because she did not want to worry me, because we are past the point of being able to control anything, but not yet at the point where we can *know*. This awful, strange, in-between room. I am torn between a desire to have my fears allayed, or postponed, at least, and a desire to have them confirmed, *now*, once and for all, so that I can move forward. Until the scan, though, it's guesswork. It *could* be a miscarriage. It *could* even be nothing, though the likelihood of this seems to be diminishing with every hour. I find myself hoping it is just a miscarriage. *Hoping! Just!* I hardly recognise myself. But I turn another page in my book and the thought, the feeling, is still there: I am afraid for myself, right now, and myself only.

A sinking suspicion, then, but without proof, you carry on. After the doctor says I can go home, call if anything changes, here's our twenty-four-hour line, I walk to the bus stop, thinking about what to cook for dinner – it's late so something easy, perhaps I'll pick up some fishcakes from the Tesco Metro on the way home. Alexander meets me at the bus stop, frustrated by traffic, but, I think, what difference really would it have made for him to be there with me, at the hospital, doing nothing much but waiting, and staring at my shoes, and turning the creamy pages of my book over and over in that terrible in-between room?

So we go home. We eat dinner. We watch an episode of *Game of Thrones*. The next day, a Saturday, we plough ahead with errands and social engagements as if nothing at all is amiss. I have a hen party in the evening, for the friend who's getting married in September, and so I put on a black dress and very high heels. I brush my hair and flick mascara onto my eyelashes. Red lipstick, no coat, it's not necessary on such a mild night. In the mirror I look like myself: not pale, not ill or off, not even very tired. As I walk around the corner to my friend's house I find myself evaluating the pain, the likelihood that something is seriously wrong. With each step that I take during which I can feel no pain I think, *well, maybe it's all right after all. Maybe it's in my head, maybe it's nothing, maybe maybe maybe . . .* and then when, occasionally, the pain asserts itself I think, *but still, it might be nothing.* And all the while some deeper hum inside me is droning, *who are you kidding?*

At my friend's house the other women are already gathered; it's a small group, just four of us in total, drinks and dinner and that's it, no funny business, no strippers, no sashes, no shots. They are sipping prosecco and I accept a glass but demur when a top-up is offered. Eventually I have to give an excuse, or perhaps I don't, but in any case I say something stupid, like, oh, I have these blood tests tomorrow, I don't feel like I should drink too much. Do they notice? Do they buy it? Does it matter? But I think: I cannot say what the truth is, because I do not know, because I do not have the words, because the outcome has not been decided yet.

A part of me remembers thinking this two years ago, the first time I miscarried. Two of these women were there with me, walking in the winter dusk, and perhaps I should know better now. But also I think: when you're celebrating your impending marriage, do you really want to think about things like this? Do you want to have someone explain the mechanics of ovulation and fertilisation and fallopian tubes?

And then I think: is it her or myself I'm protecting? The truth is it's easier, by which I mean easier for me, to pretend everything is normal. Perhaps I even start to believe it: that nothing is wrong, or nothing much, anyway. That this is just another Saturday night, just another hen do; that *this*, this feeling, this fear, this shock of pain, there one moment, gone the next, is just a blip, just one of those inexplicable things, that it will resolve itself, perhaps in the morning, perhaps if I just forget about it I will wake up and find myself cured.

On Sunday we go for lunch with some friends who live on a narrowboat. It is a soft August day and they have pulled their kitchen table from the boat and set it up on a strip of grass between the towpath and the river so that we can sit outside. Everything is normal except that nothing is normal. Eating roast lamb and salad I start to feel woozy, unsteady, but probably, I reason, it's just the movement of the boat beside me, bobbing on a river current: I am seasick, anxious, that is all. *Do I feel well in myself?* Yes. No. Maybe. Maybe not. In early evening we drive to the hospital for the blood test, where we have to wait a few extra hours because the senior doctor on call is delivering a baby by emergency C-section and the junior doctor wants her opinion before sending me home for the night. We have not brought any supplies for such a wait; neither of us has a book, or a full phone battery, so we sit and stare at the waiting room floor, then the waiting room walls, then the waiting room ceiling. We read all of the leaflets, all of the posters, all of the advertisements for medical studies, all of the numbers for helplines and URLs for charitable organisations that promise to offer support during difficult times. We watch the unmanned reception desk as if someone might suddenly appear, as if it is not a strange Sunday night in the height of the summer holidays, as if this is just a routine appointment.

When the senior doctor finally comes down, in scrubs, with a harried expression, a rushed apology, I look at her hands. Not that long ago, I think, perhaps only moments ago, those hands were literally delivering a baby. And now what? They are pressing my abdomen, in which there is nothing, or nothing much, or perhaps something, but in the wrong place. They are taking my pulse. They are opening a file, flipping through it. And then, with the usual caveat, that if I start to feel ill, or dizzy, if the pain or the bleeding gets worse, then I should come back to the hospital immediately, without delay, don't phone first, just show up, she sends me home, this woman who has just delivered a baby.

On the way home, because we promised we would, before we knew that my appointment would take several hours, we pay a visit to Alexander's dying grandfather, who is in a care home not far from the hospital. The last time I will ever see him, as it turns out: eleven o'clock at night, the air humid and sweet. We sign ourselves in to the home, even though no one checks the log. We squeeze antibacterial hand gel into our palms and the smell briefly washes away all the other smells, the pallid food, the dying, the forgetting, the old boiled wool, the disinfectant, the fresh flowers that someone brought. Alexander's grandfather, not a large man to begin with, has shrunk almost to invisibility, buried beneath layers and layers of blankets, cold even on this mild August evening, even in this overheated room. There's classical music playing, a tune we can't quite pick out – familiar somehow, but far away, something from an old film, perhaps. A single lamp glows weakly. Very little is said, apart from some commentary on the music – *do you recognise this? It's, um* . . . Alexander holds his grandfather's hand for a while; his mother is in France, has asked us to let her know whether she needs to cut the trip short to be with her father. I sit on the edge of a wooden chair, a few feet away from the bed, smiling and making soothing gestures and worrying pointlessly about the blood test results, which now indicate, definitively, that the pregnancy is not proceeding normally, although nothing else can be known until the scan on Tuesday. I force myself back into the room: it is not fair to bring my own worries here; what good can they do anyone in this place, what good for that matter can they do me? For a moment I almost see, sitting on the edge of my chair, that the moment, this moment, and then the next, is all we ever have, all we ever will have, any of us, from birth until death, and that is no small thing. Almost.

In the silences a small clock, positioned on the bedside table, ticks audibly, though its face is hidden by shadows.

Before we go the night nurse ushers us into his office and tells us that he's been doing this for a long time, and he can tell when someone is ready to go, and that Alexander's grandfather, in spite of his frailty, his skeletal form, isn't quite there yet.

(He's right, as it turns out: there are still a few weeks of life left.) What can we do? On the way home we stop by a petrol station and buy an oven pizza that we warm and then pick at, half-heartedly, before bed.

4

Tender

We have a full day before the scan: a lost day. On Monday morning Alexander calls the office to say he won't be coming into work. I do the same, claiming illness, which is true in a way, though I feel fine. But then we don't know what to do, how to be. Somehow we make time pass and then in the evening we go for a walk. On our way home we run into one of my colleagues and his wife, also out for a walk. I feel embarrassed, I'm so clearly not ill, out walking with my husband, wearing shorts and a T-shirt, sunglasses pushed onto my head. I feel as if I should explain, or justify my absence. But what could I possibly say, in passing? How could I explain, when I hardly understand myself? I'm both pregnant and not pregnant, I might say. I'm not ill but I could become ill, in fact it could kill me, this state of sort-of-pregnancy, but on the other hand I don't know anything for certain, all I have are some blood tests, two faded lines on a strip of paper: the story hasn't been written yet.

The scan, of course, shows an empty uterus, because the embryo is elsewhere – lodged in the left fallopian tube, its presence signalled only by a faint 'bagel-shaped' bulge, a common if subtle indicator. Now, after weeks of hesitation, things move quickly: I'm scheduled for surgery that afternoon, a salpingectomy, during which they will remove my entire left fallopian tube, reducing the possibility that anything unwanted might be left behind. A doctor prints off wristbands for me and inserts a cannula into the thick vein at the side of my right wrist. I look at her feet when I start to feel the pressure in my wrist; she's wearing ballet flats, a knee-length skirt, her legs are bare. I'm given a private room by the devastatingly beautiful young nurse I met when I was here earlier in the year, after my second miscarriage, for a D&C. 'No offence, but I hope I never see you here again!' she'd said to me cheerfully then – a thing, I've learned, they all say. 'Me too!' I'd said, even though the anaesthetic and the richness of her voice and the darkness of her hair had made me a little bit in love with her.

I can't get over how *nice* everyone is being, how accommodating, how understanding. Isn't it exhausting for them? I think. Isn't it depressing? And yet somehow I am made to feel as if I am the only patient on the ward, the only person in the world who matters. I am made to feel as if it might, in spite of everything, be all right in the end.

Sitting on the edge of the bed, typing out a few quick emails to cancel meetings, waiting to be told when to change into my gown and stockings, it occurs to me that this might change our story in quite drastic ways – not least because losing a fallopian tube reduces your chances of conceiving naturally – but also that, for a moment at least, I don't care, I don't even have to care: for now I just want to be OK. I just want to go for a swim, have a beer in the garden, feel the sun on my face, plan a trip somewhere.

As the anaesthetist puts me under we talk about where I'm from. 'California,' he says. 'Good wine there.' I close my eyes and picture a glass of Pinot Noir, a hummingbird, a sliver of ocean on the horizon.

After the surgery I swim around in a fentanyl- and general anaesthetic-induced haze for a few hours. 'Are you OK? You've been staring at that wall for forty minutes,' Alexander says eventually. He looks worried, or I think he does, though I can't seem to focus my eyes on his familiar face, the hazel eyes, the beard, the skin I feel I know better than my own. In that moment I can hardly speak, let alone articulate how deeply, profoundly compelling the painting across from my bed is, even though later I won't remember anything about it except that it was a sort of pastoral landscape – a field of wheat, perhaps, the undulance of a green hill in the background, an oak tree shading the foreground. *I'm looking at the painting*, I say, or try to say, or think, at least. Someone brings me a cheese sandwich and a plastic cup full of juice, but my throat is too sore from the endotracheal tube to manage more than half the sandwich. Then it's midnight and Alexander is going home, because no visitors are allowed overnight, and I am alone in the room, the lights dimmed. I am woozy and wired, so I watch the Olympics on my phone: heat after heat of the women's 800 metres; Jason Kenny doing lap after lap of the track in an apparently unending men's keirin final that they have to restart twice. Repetitive, circular sports, which soothe me into a kind of dreamless sleep, interrupted every few hours by a nurse who comes to check my blood pressure. When I wander down the hallway to pee, the ward seems empty and silent – no evidence of other patients, no sounds except mechanical ones: beeps, clicks, ticks, tocks.

In the morning a doctor comes to see me and then I am discharged, just like that. She examines the three incisions they have made, two very small and one, low on my pelvis, a bit bigger. Of the smaller ones she says they will heal quickly, that the stitches will dissolve in time. When she comes to the third incision, the bigger one, which had begun to seep a bit after the surgery and which is covered with gauze, she winces and says: and that one, well, you'll just have to be a bit patient. It will heal when it heals. They give me leaflets and pills and instructions that I immediately forget, thank God Alexander is back, listening and retaining the information that is passing through me as if I'm a sieve. Gingerly I extract myself from the hospital gown, pull my sweatpants over the compression stockings that it seems like too much trouble to remove. Alexander carries my bag and my leaflets and my pills to the car. He drives slowly, flinching at every speed hump and roundabout and red light while I sit very still, not exactly in pain but assailed by a sense of tenderness and fragility. I have the sense that were I to make any sudden movements, to sit up straight or forget my compromised position for a moment, I might dissolve or break apart, though I know the human body is not as delicate as all that.

At home Alexander sets me up in bed. Pillows, a glass of water, painkillers, my phone in case I need anything. Then he goes downstairs to putter around the house; I hear the kitchen door open, the sound of the radio, of the kettle whistling, of floorboards creaking. In the afternoon he brings me a cheese and tomato sandwich with foamy white bread, which I have requested specifically. I mostly sleep, and when I wake I get up and walk the length of the upstairs corridor to try to keep my circulation going, my heart beating, my brain moving.

Dignity is impossible to preserve: this isn't what we signed up for when we met, I think, catching a glimpse of myself in the hall mirror, looking quickly away. I think of who we were, the two of us at that pub late on a summer evening, my low-cut shirt, his soft brown blazer, the way we looked, fresh-faced even the next morning, after too much cider, too much gin, the promise of the meeting. The start of something. You don't tend to think, at the start of something, of who it will cause you to become – only of what you are now, what you might like to be. And now what? I am minus one internal organ. My belly is distended because of the gas they used to inflate my abdominal cavity for surgery, my back is hunched because it hurts to straighten up, my hair hasn't been brushed in two days, nor my teeth, I am still wearing the compression stockings under my baggy sweatpants, my breasts are sagging under a too-tight

T-shirt. This wasn't the plan, the path, the place we meant to find ourselves.

But then again: isn't it exactly what we signed up for? Isn't it exactly what a marriage, or any long-term relationship, is? What a family is?

5

A Different Story

I think I have felt, for years now – ever since the elation of those first heady months of 'trying', before it felt like trying, when every new period felt like a possibility, not a punishment, when a baby felt truly just around the corner – that I have been essentially alone on this journey. At times – often – I have excluded even Alexander, who is integral to the story: I have pushed him away, or overlaid his needs with my own. I have taken succour from the assurances of friends and acquaintances only when it has suited me, only when I feel that their words or their actions adequately match up to my own anguish or my own anger. Mostly I have chosen not to speak too much, to minimise the impact of every wound, both great and small, and in my head to write my own version of a story in which the world is actively against me, in which the scowls of other women lost in their own dramas are in fact directed at me, in which I am always moving, unwittingly, unwantingly, against the great tide of everyone else.

It would be disingenuous now to continue to spin out that narrative. Instead there are a thousand kindnesses, a thousand mercies, that come to me in flashes after the surgery. Complete strangers offer themselves up like old friends, even though they owe me nothing: the nurse who rings a few days after the surgery to check that I'm OK. I know how disorienting it can be, she says. She gives me her mobile number. If you ever need to talk . . . The doctor who visits me the morning I'm discharged. Do you remember me? she says. I saw you last week. I just wanted to come and see how you're doing. The night nurse, summoned by a bell, who gives me some codeine for the pain and then, just as she's about to leave, looks at me suddenly and says, this happened to me, too, when I was younger, and now, look, I'm OK! Later Alexander tells me that while I was in surgery he went to get himself a coffee and in the lobby he ran into someone he plays football with whose wife, it turns out, also had an ectopic pregnancy last year. These stories, these kindnesses, these mercies and moments, are everywhere.

I see them. I hear them.

6

The Resilience of the Body

There are a lot of ways to blame your body – yourself – for what does not go right. That cigarette you had one night with a friend in the pub garden. Those glasses of wine at dinner. The weed you smoked at college, the cocaine you shouldn't have accepted but did, the pressure you put yourself under to pass an exam or write a thesis, the anxiety you didn't want to feel but couldn't help, the antidepressants you were on, and then weren't on, and then were on again, and then were off, for good, for better or worse. Little things: the swim you skipped; the swim you didn't. Big things: the way you were born, the way you were built, the unconscious, unseen things that happen underneath the skin. Whose responsibility is it, other than yours? *Perhaps you should try this, or try that,* people suggest, usually meaning, and not unkindly: there must be something you can do. Or, more precisely: there must be something *you* can do. And indeed I have thought it too: there must be something I can do. A trick, a fix. A cause. A closure.

Maybe there is, or maybe there's just luck, chance, correlation without causation. No one can quite say.

At one point, after my second miscarriage, I remember going for a run. It had been an unproductive work day, a day that felt like running into a solid wall again and again. I forced myself outside and started moving my arms and my legs, not really making any conscious decision to do so, following one of my usual routes around the city, up a hill, down broad, bland avenues. As the run started to get hard, I thought to myself: *I should enjoy this, because I can do it*, only not quite so kindly. What I actually thought to myself, as my legs were starting to deaden and my lungs to burn, was more like: *good, make it hurt, you deserve to make it hurt*. Because what good are you? What *use*?

But a thing happens, in the aftermath of the ectopic pregnancy, which is unexpected: a kind of unfurling. A forgiving. The something-you-can-do-chorus in my own head considers, for a day or two after I am home from the hospital and the drugs have worn off, the possibility of fault: it was the clomifene, it was the summer cold I had, it was the stress I was under at work, with my PhD. And then it goes silent, since none of those things can any more account for what has happened than can blind bad luck.

Strange to say, in fact, but in the period after the surgery I feel almost light-hearted: because I have my body back, because it is getting, with each day, noticeably *better*; one afternoon I walk around the block, the next twice as far; the next all the way into town. I browse eBay and bid on silk blouses and soft jumpers to wear in the coming autumn, I sit outside in the garden with a cup of coffee, I observe the late-summer flowering of the white rose we planted earlier this year, the scent of the rosemary when you brush its spines. What I don't know, what I can't reconcile (*why, what next*) weighs heavy, but in the immediate aftermath, at least, I feel my body to be wholly *mine*. I enjoy the gentle recuperative swims that I am, once the stitches dissolve, allowed to take, the effects of the wine at a friend's birthday, the hours of dancing unselfconsciously at a wedding. I do not think to punish my body, or to discipline it. At the wedding, I sit next to one of the other bridesmaids, who is eight months pregnant, and I do not feel a thing except perhaps sympathy for her, with her stretched-tight polka-dot dress, her swollen ankles. Later I stand outside talking to a couple I know only a little; 'I recently had a health scare,' he says, gesturing to the vape pen that has supplanted the usual cigarette. 'We're so grateful to the NHS,' she adds. 'Everyone was so amazing.'

'They are so amazing!' I say. I want to tell them that I know this intimately. I want to say, a few weeks ago they more or less saved my life and now here I am! But instead I clink glasses with the couple and swallow a large sip of champagne.

I surprise myself, too, with a newfound devotion to my PhD. It's not so much that it gives me purpose but that it gives me, well, *something to do.* A way to spend time. As simple as that. It is the predictability, the shape it gives my days, the rhythm settling into something coherent, a melody, almost. My contract at the office ends a few weeks after the surgery, and as the three little scars heal, harden, fade, as the summer tips into autumn, I take something like pleasure in walking to the library, sitting close to a window, and attacking whatever problems my thesis – growing, growing, grown almost now to full size – presents to me each day.

I spend a lot of time in the Radcliffe Science Library, where the geography books are housed; first I descend into the dank basement, with its flickering yellow light, its smell of damp and despair, and collect heavy armfuls of texts that I think might help me make sense of what I'm writing. And then I haul myself upstairs to find a suitable desk, looking out towards the Natural History Museum. Little placards on the wall offer a word of warning – 'asbestos behind these walls' – and I take to calling this the Asbestos Library, breathing shallowly as I work until I forget to care. The knowledge that everything I am doing is in the service of a single task becomes soothing. True, it is now, suddenly, late autumn, the nights drawn out, the days dusky and muted, ready for their winter disappearance, but there is something giddy about the wind, and in the quietude of the library I find myself losing – or rather giving, without resistance or resentment – whole hours, during which nothing else can reach me, to that task.

Sometimes, during the long afternoons, I get up to stretch my legs; I roll my head from side to side, massage my shoulders, even though it feels like a very long time since I last swam hard enough to make them ache; I go to the bathroom. Before I button my jeans I trace the biggest scar, lowest down, which marks the place from which my tube was actually extracted: a permanent absence, emphasising the tenderness of flesh, the resilience – but also the rigid materiality – of the body, which must always be two things at once: what we desire and what it is in spite of desire.

A hard rain falls outside, the windows streaked. The leaves are turning, have turned, the branches are bare, the streetlights are lit, the air has a bite. I am not sure what path I am on any longer, but for the moment it seems clear and straight, and I am here.

*

It would be nice, but too easy, to say: and that was that. The stitches fell out, the scars healed, and, while I was marked by the experience, it gave me something like the courage for forgiveness, some sense, once and for all, of not being alone. Too neat, too tidy. The truth is hard and messy and full of moments of doubt and fear.

Moments like this: a few months after the surgery, after the recovery, I become convinced that it's happening again. A pain in my side, faint but persistent, a week or so before my period is due. This is the first month we've had unprotected sex since the operation and I feel instantly stupid: we shouldn't have done it, even though it was only the once, even though the next morning I went out and bought more condoms; I'm not ready to go through this again, I think, all the uncertainty, the worry, what were we thinking? I become so convinced that somehow that one night has led to another ectopic pregnancy that I call a friend of ours, a GP, and ask him what I should do. He is gentle and patient and conciliatory: even if it *is* what I fear, it's extremely unlikely I would be able to feel symptoms yet, and the probability is anyhow almost absurdly small.

That weekend we're due to fly to France, to stay with Alexander's parents at the house in Brittany they have recently bought and renovated. November; one of the last flights of the season, a skip over the Channel, a swoop into Dinard. In spite of the reassurances of our GP friend I am still anxious; any trust I had built up in my own understanding of my body has dissolved, and been replaced by a ferocious mistrust that doesn't answer to logic or reason. When we land I immediately look up where the nearest hospital is, just in case. I start to feel dizzy. A symptom? A symptom, surely, I decide. In the giant Leclerc, shopping for wine for dinner, I'm overcome with wooziness. I don't feel well at all, I tell Alexander, and go to sit in the car while his parents finish their shopping, wondering at what point I have to swallow my pride and call it a crisis.

But then we drive down to the sea, to a long, wide beach at the edge of dusk. We fan out on the sand, walking alongside the water. It is cold, a bright wind pinking my cheeks, and I zip up my jacket and walk and walk, stooping every so often to pick up a stone, turn it in my hand. One in particular pleases me, soothes the skin in my palm, and I place it in my pocket and hold it there, and after a while we turn back and head for home. At dinner I am still woozy but I think, fuck it, and have a few glasses of cold, sharp white wine with my *coquilles Saint Jacques,* until I can't tell the wine-wooziness from the anxiety-wooziness.

On the flight home I read while Alexander sleeps, gazing sometimes out to the blue below, and when we get into Stansted, in spite of the grimness and vastness of the car park and the long drive still ahead of us, in spite of the fact that I still have no definitive proof that I'm OK (but what would be definitive proof?), I feel lighter, light enough to sense that there might be a way through, a way out.

I think: well, maybe now I have to live with this fear always. But perhaps after all I *can* live with it.

★

Or like this: a year after the surgery, almost to the day. Another faint pain, another panic. I have actually got my period this time, but it's different, lighter than usual, I feel strange, I cannot ignore the signs I'm sure my body is giving me. I take a test – negative – but what reassurance is that really: false negatives are more common than false positives, after all, and wouldn't it be just like me, I think, to betray myself like this? It's Friday evening, before a bank holiday; we're due to go to Dorset the next morning. I call my GP surgery just before they're set to shut and the doctor I speak with tells me that if I think it would help, if I really want to rule the possibility out, the best thing, the only thing, is to go to A&E. So I do.

The doctor who eventually comes to see me, after I have been issued with wristbands at reception and led through a series of hallways to a series of waiting areas, snaps to attention before me, literally. He has a military bearing and a military rank on the name tag clipped to his scrubs. He is young and tall and preposterously handsome, like he belongs in a film. What must he think of me, this bedraggled woman, in a holey jumper and ripped jeans, talking to him about the colour and consistency of her period blood? I am ashamed, and then ashamed that I should feel this way, as if it matters.

In the end he is kinder to me than perhaps my situation warrants. 'What can I do to reassure you?' he asks. I shake my head: I don't know. He sits down on a stool, wheels it closer to me. I get the sense that he has been gauging what kind of person I am from the way that I am speaking – analytically, emotionally distant, trying to back up my irrational fears with empirical evidence – and that now he has the measure of me he is going to talk to me on my level. He sits and regards me as an equal, though even seated he is much taller than I am. I wish I had brushed my hair, put on mascara at least. Your test was negative, right? he says. I nod. If everything in medicine, he says, were as reliable as a pregnancy test, my job would be a lot easier. Sure, they're not 100 per cent, but they're pretty damn close. And so on: he talks me down from the ledge. After a while he asks if I am OK, if I feel any better. I do, in that moment. He walks with me out the door, down the corridor, so that I can find my way back to the entrance, which has been lost to me in the stress and the confusion. As we walk I apologise for wasting his time, for being silly. He laughs, and I see for a moment that what to me is a significant event, a terrifying, embarrassing moment, is to him nothing at all, just business as usual; he won't remember me in a few hours, let alone tomorrow, next week, next year. Look, he says, it's a Friday night in A&E: at least you haven't tried to punch me or insulted my mother!

Still I spend the drive down to Dorset the next morning constantly evaluating my symptoms, in spite of the reassurance of the good-looking doctor, in spite of the evidence. Is that pain indicative of something? What do I really feel? Even when we meet up with our friends at the campsite, put up tents, still I am thinking always of this fear, still at the back of my mind is this doubt, this dread. But it's a hot bank holiday Saturday and now we are on a beach, and now we are in the water, which is cold and blue-green in the mid-afternoon light, a slight wind giving it chop, and later, sitting on a grassy hill, drinking cider, I confess to my friend that last night I visited A&E, and while it is embarrassing, it is also good to say, and over the weekend, with each swim, the fear fades a little.

It fades, and goes on fading, even if it will never be gone.

7

The Habits of a Landscape

I have begun to see my scars as a sort of inscription. They have been cut into me; they have meaning, weight. They are saying something.

An inscription, the anthropologist Sally Ann Ness writes, *preserves its meaning by sinking deeply into an unchanging place.* For a moment I feel something fearful, reading that: *sinking*, so antithetical to the idea of swimming, or floating, or thriving; *unchanging*, when all I want is to change, to see that change, that swell of breasts and belly, and anyway what place is ever truly unchanging? But there's something alluring about it. Sinking deeply: perhaps unexpected things can become anchors, rather than weights.

Sometimes in the changing room at the pool, when I am completely naked after my shower, before I have slipped on my bra and my underpants and my T-shirt and my jeans and become again the outside version of myself, as I am rubbing lotion on my legs or deodorant under my arms, I wonder if these marks are visible. Some of the women here, it occurs to me, might even themselves know what they mean. One of them, I know, is a nurse; perhaps she can read them, the three tiny lines, perhaps she has seen them before.

But they are very small, after all, and mostly I have my back to the other women while I am changing, and even if they could see, even if they did understand, what then, what would I want them to say, to do? Is it not true that the greatest comfort in coming here is in the resistance and submission of the water, yes, but also in smiling and nodding at the faces I recognise, being treated as one of them, one of the regulars, someone who belongs, just another woman? Who here cares or even knows if I have a baby or not, if I ever will. They all have their own stories too, and if I listen sometimes I catch the edge of them, as perhaps they catch the edge of mine, and even if all we have in common is a time, a place, that's something, that's something quite substantial.

When I first became deeply involved with the pool, when I first started to go obsessively, when I joined a triathlon club, swam six days out of seven, I used to look at myself in the mirror and see a *swimmer*: I saw the pool written in the muscles in my arms, my back, felt it in the effortlessness of my stroke. When I lost that fitness I saw it as a kind of failure, I felt that I was losing myself, that *myself* was tied so closely to the pool, the habit and ritual of it, that my very shape had come to reflect this relation-ship. But now I see that perhaps there are softer, more nuanced ways for a body and a place to get along. I remember something that happened a few years ago, when I was in California for Christmas. It was eighty degrees out, a heatwave, a drought, the hills already bleached gold, a sign of profound thirst, presaging summer wildfires. I decided to go for a swim on Christmas Eve; I drove south along the 101, to the pool where my grandmother had bought me temporary membership, knowing that I wanted to continue to do my laps while I was visiting.

When I arrived there was only one other swimmer ploughing up and down, and as I approached I recognised immediately the stroke of my grandmother, on one of her own regular swims. We said hello, and then continued on our separate journeys, sharing the pool for a while, until she got out, and I had it all to myself, and I did a few lengths of backstroke, gazing upwards at the sky, letting my mind wander. I was happy to have seen my grandmother here, happy that we were the only people, seemingly, who had thought on the morning of Christmas Eve to drive to the pool and go for a swim. But now I think in particular of how I had known it was her, of how I had seen the distinctive stroke, acquired after decades of practice, marked and adjusted by time and advancing years, and known.

In her book Ness, the anthropologist, applies the idea of inscription to dance. She describes, for example, a particular movement term developed by the modern dancer and choreographer Martha Graham: the 'contraction', in which the abdominal cavity is hollowed out, with the pelvis tucked and the spine curving forward. (Its corollary is the 'release', whereby the body returns to its 'normal' state, either in a relaxed way or via an outward propulsion of energy; the cycle between contraction and release is based on the breath, with the contraction being associated with the exhale and the release with the inhale.) Dancers must practise this movement over and over again to master it, making hundreds of repetitions on a daily basis. After years of this, years of daily repetition, the movement begins to 'mark' the dancer's musculature. It is said to be 'inscribed' into the dancer's body *once the body's connective tissues themselves bear the evidence of that practice*: a kind of literal rewriting of the body.

In this account, Ness is particularly interested in the word 'in', the prefix of *inscription* – *it is a place-seeking, not a place-being, 'in'*, not, she says, the in of 'inside', but 'into'. *Inscriptive gestures*, she writes, *can be thought of as gestures that write something into a place*, where a place may be a body, a particular muscle or ligament.

Reading this I instinctively picture hard things, solid fleshy firm things: muscle, bone, a band of gold or silver, a path on a hillside, formed over the course of many years by many feet, both human and animal. The path becomes particular. There are many such paths where I grew up, paths just wide enough to accommodate a single-file line of cattle as they migrate from one end of the property to another. Whenever I visit home I find myself on one or another of them, retracing my childhood steps, very sure, although certain elements of the landscape have shifted – trees felled, rocks tumbled, brush thickened – of my footing and my route. From a distance they look like very old scars, cut across thick, tough flesh. Up close they feel like an indelible part of the earth; it is hard to imagine the place without them, before them, or what my routes might look like if they were differently positioned, even though they are not static.

(Bachelard: *And what a dynamic, handsome object is a path! How precise the familiar hill paths remain for our muscular consciousness!*)

Whenever I find myself on one of these trails I think of what Robert Macfarlane once wrote about paths, that they are *the habits of a landscape*, a phrase which seems to give some agency to landscape, as if it, too, is rooted in routine and ritual. Which I suppose to a certain extent it is: what is a path if not a manifestation of repetition? And something happens when we repeat ourselves in the same places over and over again, something like the inscriptive process that Ness describes. A place, a path, a cut is made, but so is a person: *Through living in it, the landscape becomes a part of us, just as we are a part of it*, as Tim Ingold writes.

Is this it, I think, the proof that I have lived in this landscape, this strange place that I entered what, four years ago now, the land of almost, of maybe?

Yes, say it: this place, this here, this now, has marked me. The doubt has marked me, the fear has marked me, the hope has marked me.

J.D. Dewsbury: *Landscape can change the body encountering it, which is to say that the body never leaves the field of a landscape the same as it enters it.*

8

A Breath of Wind

Four months after the surgery, in December, I'm scheduled for an appointment with a consultant: a kind of debrief, an opportunity to ask questions like *what now?* I am due to submit my PhD thesis later that week and then, a few days later, to fly out to California for a month. It feels auspicious, all these threads being wrapped up, all these new possibilities opening out.

We arrive at the hospital on a cold weekday morning, unravel ourselves in the waiting room, scarves, coats, hats. We have met the consultant before, she was the one who confirmed my second miscarriage, who ordered the MRI, with whom I have been in touch, intermittently, for many months now. She is kind and brusque in equal measure, patient and apologetic but very direct, which I appreciate – there is no point pussyfooting around things now, if there ever was.

Of course we want to know why this happened. Is it connected to the miscarriages? Just a fluke? And of course no one can say, least of all her: look, she says, sometimes these things just happen, and we don't know why, and we'll never know why. She looks tired as she says this and I imagine her having to say it over and over again to people, having to force them, over and over again, to meet the edge of what's possible to understand. I think about her sometimes, in the months after, think about how strange it must be to have so much knowledge, and yet so little. Imagine being a doctor, with many years of training and many years of hard, practical experience, a high-level consultant, a Miss or a Mister, a surgeon, a researcher, and having to shrug and to say, *it's difficult to know,* by which of course you mean it's impossible to know, you don't know, no one knows. To be reduced to platitudes, or open-ended ifs: wouldn't it wear you down?

The good news, she says, is that losing a fallopian tube doesn't cut your chances of conceiving naturally in half; if the other tube is healthy the likelihood can still be good. Then she says she'd like to do what's known as a lap-and-dye test, a laparoscopic operation where a dye is used to check whether a fallopian tube is blocked. Doing this will allow us to know for sure whether my remaining tube is functional or not. She'll put me on the list, I should get a letter in the next few months with an appointment date. In the meantime, she says, if I do become pregnant, of course she would be happy to see me, to make sure I get an early scan, all I need to do is ring her assistant, here's the number.

It shakes me a little, that appointment. I don't know what I had expected, I suppose I must have known that there would be no answers, no *definitely this, definitely not that,* no guarantees or diagnoses, but I think I had hoped to leave feeling lighter than when I went in, and instead I am burdened by a new set of considerations. On our way home Alexander and I stop for a coffee. I stir a cube of sugar into my latte. Another surgery. I think about the recovery process in August: oh, I felt better and better every day, but it was three weeks before I felt *myself,* and much longer still before I felt I could shake the fear. Do I want to go through that again – even a milder version, less traumatic, less invasive? Do I want to walk into a hospital well and emerge wounded? But I am being offered something that I have spent years seeking, chasing, desiring: more knowledge. If the remaining tube is patent, then it is still possible for me to conceive naturally, it still might happen just as we thought it would at the start. If it isn't, then we'll be eligible immediately for an NHS-funded cycle of IVF. Even if it is, I'll still become eligible for an NHS-funded cycle of IVF if we don't conceive within two years of the ectopic pregnancy, assuming the rules don't change between now and then.

Either way I'll know more than I know now. Either way I can't control the outcome.

*

Six months later, I get a letter, with an appointment date in two weeks' time. When I arrive it is like before, and before that, and before that. A nurse takes me to a curtained-off cubicle where she takes my vitals and asks me a series of questions, starting with my name and date of birth. When she asks if I have had any other surgical procedures, I shrug and say, nothing that isn't in my file, and she looks at me with her head tilted and says: why don't you tell me. Assume I know nothing. So I tell her. I start at the beginning. I want to say, *it's all there, in that file you're holding*, but instead I trace the journey: well, I say, I've been here before . . .

Before I'm asked to change into my gown, the consultant we met with in December stops by to speak with me, to reiterate what the procedure is, what they are looking for. After the procedure I am wheeled to a bay on the ward, a thin plastic curtain separating me from the other women; I can hear their voices, one next to me complaining of pain, while across the aisle a girl in her late teens is asking the nurse questions on behalf of her mother, who is still woozy from the anaesthetic and whose English is not as good as her daughter's. I myself feel OK; I do not have the urge to stare at a wall, fall into a painting, I'm eager to drink the tea and eat the sandwich and get on with my evening. I feel hardly any pain at all.

After about an hour the consultant stops by to tell me how it went: everything looks good! she says. Perhaps in my drowsy state I have imagined the exclamation mark, have projected a false inflection onto her, but to me it seems as if she herself is happy for me, can't wait to share the news. She opens a file and shows me some photographs taken during the procedure. So this is how it is, I think: even when you *see* your own insides, you don't really understand. The photos mean nothing to me, partly because I'm not a doctor, and partly because I'm high on general anaesthetic, pain meds, and relief. They look like orangey-pink abstract images, like the kind of photo you get when you accidentally take a close-up of your own finger with your phone. They look like alien landscapes, like topographical maps of another planet, which in a way I suppose they are, this strange planet of my body, the interior life of it, the inner workings that no one quite understands.

A few days before the procedure, towards the end of our holiday, we had walked up Snowdon, in Wales; a long slog up, for which we were rewarded by a dense fog obscuring any view from the top, and then right back down the way we'd come. On the way down I remembered how on our honeymoon two years before, climbing hill after hill in various national parks, I'd had the thought that hiking up and down hills, mountains, is just like swimming laps, in a way: the repetition of footfall, the going back on yourself. A pilgrimage, a ritual, a way of knowing, of being in a body. The terrain here was different – dark puffy clouds, puddles and stiles and stone walls – but the feeling of it, the rhythm of it, called me back to other landscapes. And what was different now? Nothing, but everything.

For the whole holiday, but on that hike in particular, I was preoccupied by worry about the surgery, small as it was. I felt the fear of losing something – of losing fitness, ground, vitality – of being cast back into the role of patient, even if briefly, of feeling weak, compromised, feeling as if my body were misbehaving. Perhaps I even felt that the me outside of the hospital was a person in the world again, but that as soon as I submitted to the cannula, to the anaesthetic, I would be again just another faulty woman. Would I say that in the last few months I had been able to effectively relax, to forget how much I still want a baby? Not exactly, but in some ways other things had momentarily superseded the desire: I had got my PhD, I had gone on holiday, I had stayed up late drinking wine and feeling the spin of the world, I had started, tentatively, to think about a career, a future.

Walking up the mountain the burn of muscles was a pleasure, so was the cold of the fog at the summit, the small blister that my boots rubbed on my toe, the smell of mud and dust and grass. When we got back to the hotel the shower was a pleasure, and the pint of lager we drank on a bench outside a pub in Beddgelert, our backs to the sun that had suddenly come out: I sat there and thought of nothing at all. On the other hand I knew that I could not stay in the dark, I knew I wanted to know what the test showed: otherwise we would just be stuck, wouldn't we, otherwise we wouldn't know how to proceed, and I wanted to proceed, I wanted to move forward.

Now, after the surgeon departs, Alexander and I are left alone for a while. I can still hear the woman on the other side of the curtain: she is uncomfortable, her back hurts, I suppose she can hear us, too, our murmurings, our news. When the nurse comes to discharge me she hands me a printout of my discharge summary. Looking at it later, at home, the giddiness of relief fading, I'm not quite sure what it is I've actually learned. My remaining tube is patent, yes, but what does that mean, what does that guarantee? A door has been left open for me, perhaps – that's all it is.

Even so, now we can proceed; this is a step forward. A breath of wind ruffling a calm flat sea – not enough to propel us out of the doldrums, perhaps, but still, it's something. What will happen next? We don't know. Nothing is wrong with me; nothing is certain; nothing is out of the question. We still want what we want, of course, but perhaps we can allow ourselves to want other things, too. In the meantime we have options. We can pick up where we left off. We can pay for IVF as private patients, put it on a credit card, start right away. We can do nothing at all for a while, if we choose. The thing is: we *can* choose. It feels for the first time in a long time as if we have some agency, even though we know now, perhaps better than most, that we have no control at all over the outcome of our choice.

A month or so later, we go for a walk along the river. We walk to the pub, the same pub where we made our first decision, four years ago, or was it a lifetime? We order drinks, sit outside even though the sky suggests rain. Another decision: we'll see what happens. It's been almost exactly a year since the ectopic pregnancy. If I don't conceive in the next year, we'll be able to claim our free cycle of IVF. What's another year, at this point? In some ways it's a lot: a lot of time, a lot still unresolved. But in other ways it's not so much; the time will not be wasted, irresolution is not always the end of the world, in fact sometimes it's a world of its own. For now, at least, we'll just wait and see what happens.

Six

A Bright Spot

2018–

I

Reconciliation

Time passes, as it always does, in a rush and a blur, at least retro-spectively. How can it be that already the shops are decorated for Halloween, now for Christmas, it feels like New Year's Day was only yesterday, how can I be another year older already – thirty, thirty-one?

In the summer of 2018, two years after the ectopic pregnancy, we become eligible for an NHS-funded round of IVF. In those years it has always been at the back of my mind that I might conceive naturally – although the loss of my left fallopian tube has reduced my chances it has not, as the doctors have been very keen to tell me, even halved them, and there are no other obvious impediments to conception. But the IVF deadline has also given us a curious freedom. We can wonder whether I am ovulating on any given day, or we can forget about that for a while. We can *try*, but we don't have to. We can get on with other things, safe in the knowledge that, if nature does not take its course, we can hand the responsibility over to someone else in a year or two.

In order to receive our funding we have to attend an appointment with a doctor, who looks through our paperwork and confirms our eligibility. There are also numerous tests to undergo – blood tests, semen analysis, all things we have done on multiple occasions before, but everything must be up to date. When we receive the official confirmation of our funding, in September, we are excited. We make an appointment at the clinic as quickly as we can.

A long protocol cycle of IVF, we learn at the appointment, involves a number of phases. First, during the 'down regulation' phase, you suppress your natural cycle via medication – in my case, a nasal spray that I will administer twice a day for several weeks, in the morning and the evening, tilting my head back afterwards and tasting a sharpness at the back of my throat, the only real evidence I have that anything at all is happening. Once your cycle has been suppressed, you begin to inject yourself daily with what's called follicle stimulating hormone, to increase the number of eggs your ovaries produce. The more eggs the better, to a point, though there's also a risk of over-stimulation, which can be dangerous and counter-productive. Your progress during the stimulation phase, which usually lasts somewhere between ten and twelve days, is assessed via regular scans to monitor your ovaries and note the number and quality of the developing eggs. About thirty-six hours before your eggs are due to be collected, you take a precisely timed 'trigger injection', a final shot of hormones to help the eggs mature. During the egg collection itself you are sedated while a doctor passes a needle through the vagina and into each ovary. The extracted eggs are then mixed with the donor or partner sperm in the lab. After between sixteen and twenty hours, they're checked to see if any have fertilised. Those that have are monitored in the laboratory for up to six days; the aim is for an embryo to get to the blastocyst stage before being transferred back to the womb – in other words, for it to be as well developed as possible. Then comes the embryo transfer, done using a catheter passed into the vagina and guided by ultrasound. Then a wait of around two weeks before a pregnancy test can determine whether or not the embryo has successfully implanted. From the first sniff of the down-regulation drugs to the pregnancy test it might be something like six weeks, or longer.

There are people who find IVF to be an alarming prospect. There are people for whom this is the line they will not cross, all the injections, the hormones, the mood swings, the medicalisation of such an old human process, the artificiality of it. I can understand this, especially when the whole thing is laid out to us, from start to uncertain finish. It is a lot to take in, a lot to commit to, a lot of physical and emotional work. But I find it surprisingly easy to submit myself to the regimen. I find that I like the idea of ceding control, I like the idea of giving my body to the clinic, saying here, you take over for a while. I like the attention, all the appointments, the one-on-one conversations with doctors and nurses, the way the process of conception is abstracted by being broken down to its component parts: it does not make me feel strange but rather gives me great comfort to imagine Alexander's sperm being introduced to my eggs in a controlled, safe environment, outside the storm-racked sea of my body, where they might stand a better chance of having a productive meeting.

After we have our first consultation with our clinic, I receive in the post a thick booklet, outlining in some detail each stage of the process. I find it difficult to wrap my head around the journey as a whole; I can really only think about it one step at a time. Bits of information about what will happen further down the line keep falling from my head. At any point along the way, I think, something might go wrong, we might have to go back to the beginning again, we might discover some fatal flaw. There is no point getting ahead of ourselves.

For a long time, anyhow, we do nothing at all except wait. We cannot begin immediately, because the timing of my cycle is such that if we do, we're likely to require treatment over Christmas, when the clinic is closed. Then we have to wait another month, for my period to arrive again. By the time I start sniffing the down-regulation drugs it is December. I set alarms on my phone to remind me when to sniff. On Christmas Day I accompany my mother-in-law to church and one of the alarms goes off during a hymn; on New Year's Eve it goes off during dinner with friends and I squeeze around the table, go and stand in the lounge and tilt my head back while the medicine drips down my throat, sit back down, continue eating my Thai green curry. It feels strangely intangible, all this waiting, all this organising and keeping track of drug regimens and appointments, as if it's all a great distraction. *When will it actually begin?* I keep finding myself thinking, even though of course it already has.

On New Year's Day, early in the morning, we drive to the clinic for a scan, so that they can assess the success of the down-regulation drugs. The nurse is very pleased. Everything looks exactly as it should, she says, beaming. This is not a sentence I am used to hearing in relation to my uterus. Are you sure? we say. Oh, yes, she says. A few weeks later, we are into the stimulation phase, and things are still going well: I have a decent number of eggs developing, I am reacting just as I should be to the medication. One evening as we are making dinner Alexander turns to me and says: 'I almost don't know how to act about the fact that things are going well; I'm not used to it.'

I know what he means. I have felt us to be two shy birds, mistrustful, ready to take flight. Should we now abandon our fear, our mistrust, since the signs seem positive? Or should we hold on to it just in case? Truly we do not know what will happen, each phase is only that, a phase, with another test to pass at the end, and then another, and another. In the clinic waiting room sometimes I will glance around at the other couples and think about how so few of us will get what we really want out of this process, at least this time around; according to the Human Fertilisation and Embryology Authority, the average chance of birth from IVF treatment for women under thirty-five is 29 per cent, a figure that drops with age, to just 2 per cent for women over forty-four.[4] Whenever a scan shows that I am on track, I will realise again how unused I have become to thinking of my body as something that *behaves*, and perhaps it's strange to say but I begin almost to think of the process as a healing one, or a kind of reconciliation. I cannot abandon the fear, the mistrust, completely, but I can begin to acknowledge a new fragile faith in my body.

I am lucky, of course: I can afford to feel this way, to philosophise about it, because I do not find it too physically or emotionally taxing. Once or twice, it's true, I find myself shouting at Alexander, or breaking down in tears, out of sheer frustration: not with him, or myself, exactly, but with everything, the whole situation – what has happened to us in the past, what might or might not happen to us in the future. I feel at times as if I am not up to bearing *any* accountability for the process now; I want in effect to completely surrender my agency, let someone else be ultimately responsible for a change, and yet if I don't inject myself at exactly the right time each day, if I sneeze too soon after sniffing the down-regulation drugs, mightn't I sabotage my own chances? The pressure seems immense. How can I, who am not medically trained, possibly get everything right all the time – and still hold in my head the knowledge that even if I *do*, things still might not go my way?

The first time I have to give myself an injection my hands shake so hard I think I might have to get Alexander to do it for me, but this is impractical: with his work schedule he cannot be home every night at exactly 7 p.m. to administer each shot, and anyway when I go to hand him the syringe I suddenly realise that it would be worse, somehow, to make him do this for me, to me. I take it back and sink the needle into a pinch of skin in my stomach, and to my surprise there is no pain at all, and I think it is a small enough thing to have to do, in the grand scheme of things. By and large I find it satisfying, not stressful, to tick things off each day, to go through the motions.

On the day of the egg collection they settle me in a room and issue me with a gown to change into. While I am changing they lead Alexander away, so that he can produce his specimen of sperm in a small room down the hall.

'They have . . . *CDs* in the room,' he whispers when he comes back. 'Like, those classical music compilations you used to get free with your newspaper. And a little sign asking you to wipe everything down after.'

I picture all the other men we'd seen in the waiting room earlier that morning: I picture them putting on a Best of Bach mix and settling into an armchair. I picture them spraying the chair with disinfectant, wiping it down, placing their specimen in the hatch in the wall for a technician to collect. But nothing seems ridiculous any more. At our first consultation we'd met with a nurse who'd been working for the clinic for more than twenty years. When I first started, she'd said, we used to have to run the sperm down the hall to the lab ourselves, and I'd pictured this literally, nurses in scrubs running with glass vials of sperm, and it seemed to me that it did no good not to find something funny in all of it. But there is also a great seriousness to it: after the egg collection, during which they extract eleven eggs, we go home, and the next day an embryologist calls to tell me that nine have been fertilised, and then every day after that someone calls to give me an update on how they are developing. In the end, by day five, we have five embryos of sufficient quality. They choose one for the transfer and freeze the rest.

The transfer itself is much more straightforward than the egg collection, but afterwards I feel a strange new fragility. Can I really go about my business as usual, or should I try somehow to hold the embryo close? I feel wilfully stupid, but I can't help myself: so it's OK for me to . . . *walk around?* I ask the nurse after the procedure is finished and I am pulling up my trousers. Can I go to the bathroom now, or should I wait? She smiles understandingly. Think of it this way, she says. Picture a grain of sand in a jar of jam: it's not going to just . . . slip out. You can go to the bathroom.

I understand, I say, although I'm not sure I do. Even picturing the grain of sand in a jar of jam, it feels so delicate, so intangible: how can I possibly really understand it, I wonder, how can I wrap my head around it, my body around it?

Before we leave the nurse hands me a small packet containing a jar in which to urinate, a pregnancy test to dip into the urine, and instructions on what to do if the test is negative, what to do if the test is positive. I can't take the test for almost two weeks: another wait, another in-between room, more almost, more maybe. It requires faith, I think – not only in the outcome itself, but in your body, in your mind, in your ability not to crumble or dissolve.

Will I dissolve?

I don't know for sure, but I don't think so.

2

A Place for the Unknown

The pregnancy test, when I take it, is positive. It is early February, and snowing hard. A magical morning, the flakes large and settling thickly. I have a lecture to give, and so in the snow I trudge up the hill to campus and try to talk to my students about heritage and landscape, about the way humans have left their mark on the earth, while the bigger part of my mind wanders off, elsewhere, into a realm of possibility and potential.

Later that afternoon, squinting through snow flurries, we drive to Whitstable. We'd planned the trip before we knew what the outcome of the test would be, so that it could be either a celebration or a consolation. We arrive in an icy darkness, but in the morning it is sharply sunny, so cold that it hurts to breathe, the sea a compendium of blue-green-greys. Walking along the pebble beach I stray close to the edge of the water and lean forward to touch it, feel its fizz. It laps at my feet, over the toes of my boots, leaving a line of salt. After breakfast we drive to Margate; the roads are empty and I suck a Werther's Original to combat a touch of nausea that I can't be certain I have not imagined, or willed into being, wanting I suppose some palpable, physical sign, not just two lines on a plastic stick but something inside myself that I can grasp on to. *I won't obsess over this*, I tell myself, *I'll just take things as they come*, but I can already feel that to say this is one thing, to do it quite another.

At the Turner they have an exhibition by the Scottish artist Katie Paterson. Paterson's work is interested in scientific

240

knowledge and its limits, in geological time, deep space, in things like moonlight and melting glaciers and dead stars. The exhibition features a number of her projects, each of which, in its own way, seems to form a bridge between the staid rigour of research and the emotional pull of the Romantic sublime. In one room a mirror ball hangs from the ceiling; its surface is made of over 10,000 images of solar eclipses, from drawings hundreds of years old to recent, cutting-edge telescopic photos, which reflected in the darkness of the room look like all the stars of the universe spinning across the gallery walls. Meanwhile in the corner an automated grand piano plays Beethoven's 'Moonlight Sonata', except that it is a 'moon-altered' version of the piece: it has been translated into Morse code, sent to the moon, reflected off its surface, and received back on earth. The altered piece is recognisable but fragmented, because the moon *reflects only part of the information back: some is absorbed in its shadows or lost in its craters.* The absences, translated into rests, are felt deeply but not keenly, catching your attention but not holding it. The effect of these two pieces juxtaposed is hypnotic, almost stupefying. I feel as if I am swimming in the deep; I do not want to leave the room, and we stay for a long time, as other people come and go.

Later, on a placard, I read a statement by Paterson: *I think it's really important that there is still a place for the unknown*, she has said. She talks about the uncharted wilderness of the 'deeper universe', the places where knowledge and progress haven't yet reached. I write it down in my notebook: *The unknown point that you can't put into words.*

3

The Hard Edges

When you do IVF, they tell you not to swim or take baths until the outcome is known. They say that water can be absorbed and can interfere with the scans. When I first heard this I was alarmed, of course – all the old questions, how would I exercise, how would I maintain my sanity, my sense of control, the rootedness of routine? But the truth is I have found it easier than I thought I would to give it up, for a time. My last swim before the cycle began was unexceptional, unmemorable. Morning, a weekday. I shared a lane with two women I have got to know a bit over the years, chatted with them as we got dressed after, cycled home in cold autumn air. 'See you tomorrow!' one of the women said as I was leaving the changing room. 'Yes!' I said, but of course I wouldn't see her tomorrow, as it turned out.

For a few days I itched to get back to the pool, woke at the same time I would for a swim. But then the desire receded – and anyway now I had other rituals, other routines to occupy myself with: precisely timed sniffs of nasal spray, injections, vaginal pessaries containing progesterone to be inserted three times a day. I thought: the pool will still be there when I want it, when I'm ready for it, won't it?

★

Before we started the IVF cycle, I decided to try acupuncture. People kept recommending it to me; friends I trusted had found it transformative, or at the very least soothing. Someone sent me a link to information about a study in 2008 that suggested that acupuncture could actually increase the chances of getting pregnant for women undergoing IVF.[5] It seemed to me that I had little to lose but money, and although I was not overly keen to have someone stick needles in me, I had by now lost the squeamishness that might in earlier years have stopped me.

I booked an appointment with a fertility specialist. When I arrived for the session, eager and apprehensive in equal measure, she escorted me to the treatment room and got straight to the point. She asked me a series of questions about my diet, my periods, my bowel movements. She asked questions like: when you drink water, do you sip it, or do you glug it? (I glug it, I said. Hmmm, she said, as if this were not unexpected, but also not the healthy answer.)

After she had written some things down on her clipboard and examined the surface of my tongue, she told me that a lot of it was about what modifications I was willing to make, what sacrifices. Ask yourself, she said: what am I willing to give up for this? 'This' being a euphemism for a successful pregnancy, a baby. She said she believed firmly that diet and exercise have a huge impact on our reproductive health. She listened horrified while I told her about my exercise history: I used to love running, I said, but I've stopped for now (good, she said, running is so bad for you!). My main form of exercise is swimming, I said, but I've been advised against that for now, too. To this I got a sucking of teeth: the worst of my sins, for it might make my womb damp, and while it hasn't been proven, there's some indication that it can even cause – here I tried to stop listening, to divert the blame before it arrived, but I couldn't quite close my ears in time – complications, could be linked to ectopic pregnancies or miscarriage. I told her that I'd stopped drinking, that I'd reduced my caffeine intake: good, but not good enough – it would be better if I would forgo caffeine altogether, better in fact if I limited my consumption of all hot drinks, because it sounded like I might have a heat imbalance. And so on.

At one point she told me the story of a client who refused, she claimed, to give up her habit of drinking a bottle of wine each night. A bottle? I thought. I found this unlikely, I thought she must have either got her words wrong or else was exaggerating for effect, to make me see how simple it would be to give myself up completely: just stop drinking a bottle of wine each night! But at the end of the interrogation I nodded dumbly, I said I would take her advice. She wrote down the name of a good fertility diet book, then told me to lie back on the bed and stuck a series of needles in my arms and legs, and I tried to tune in to the sensation I knew I was supposed to be, but couldn't quite honestly claim I actually was, feeling.

'Do you feel that?' she would say, and though I could sometimes feel a pinch or a prick as the needle went in I knew that wasn't what she meant.

'Yes, I think so,' I said doubtfully.

'Sometimes it takes a few sessions,' she said.

Still: 'see you next week!' I said at the end of the session, when I'd paid my £90, and I meant it. As I went away I took with me a certain knowledge that I'd been on the wrong track the whole time: I had been trying always to be two things at once, to live two lives at once, to hedge my bets, modify my behaviour only moderately. I saw that for all these years I had not wanted to give up my habits, my routines, unless I had to, because I wanted to find a way to survive no matter the outcome, but that in so doing I had in fact merely been demonstrating a lack of commitment, perhaps even a lack of desire. This should be an act of *complete* commitment, I thought: I should want it so much that I would give everything, anything, up, should want it so much that I would give my *self* up if I had to, which in effect is what I felt was really being asked of me, to whittle myself down to a womb only, and then start again from there.

An almost catholic resolve came over me, to allow myself no transgressions, no trespasses, though it also made me itchy, uneasy, as if somewhere deep down I knew that it wasn't right.

But then later that week, after I'd spoken to Alexander, and my therapist, I found myself at dinner with some friends, telling them with mounting panic about this acupuncturist and her draconian regime: I was feeling increasingly off-kilter about the whole thing, increasingly as if the rug had been pulled out from under me. My friends, I discovered, one of whom was heavily pregnant herself, sipping a small glass of wine, were angry on my behalf: it's crazy to say that you can't have any hot drinks or that swimming might be to blame for what's gone wrong in the past, it's crazy to deprive yourself of everything, it can't be healthy. And I found myself saying, in spite of my earlier resolve, that it was true, I didn't think I could live like that, that it went against the framework I had begun trying to build for myself, this idea of balance, of a structure to govern my life that was rooted not in extremes but in allowing myself just enough freedom that I didn't accidentally stifle myself. Yes, for God's sake, they said, my friends, my husband, at least try a different acupuncturist, they're not all like that.

I did try a different acupuncturist, and when I told her I liked to swim she didn't suck her teeth, she said she did too, isn't it so helpful for anxiety? She didn't seem to care particularly what I ate. When she asked if I had read many fertility books I was honest and said no, none, that in fact I'd deliberately avoided them, because I felt it would be unhelpful to me to have too much contradictory input, or indeed to put too much stock in the idea that this or that adjustment to my diet or my sleeping habits or anything else could be the magic fix I needed, when really I knew that many things about this journey were beyond my control. She said this sounded healthy, it sounded like I had thought about it and decided what would work for me. I went to see her every week for three months, and while I don't know whether in the long term it did any good, I know it did no harm, and I found I liked our brief chats, the warmth of the room as I lay back for half an hour and went completely still.

But I wonder, even now, about the games, the denials. Complete commitment, martyrdom for a cause – do I really believe, could it really be possible, that if I pay a high enough price, give up enough, I'll be rewarded? Of course it's just another way of trying to exert control. But aren't we also really asking: *do I want it enough?* And then trying to find a way to prove that we do?

I think: perhaps I simply haven't proven it yet. Perhaps I just haven't given enough, yet.

But then I think that if we do have a baby, what kind of a mother will I be if there's nothing left of me but want for the child?

I think: to be a woman in the world is hard enough already. I must maintain some grip on myself.

A therapist once said to me: the most important thing we can do is get to know ourselves. At the time I dismissed it, I thought, well, I do know myself, I have spent more time than most analysing my actions and my foibles and my desires, I have done countless solipsistic, self-centred deep-dives into my own psyche, I write in the first person for a reason. But later, at home, I thought about it some more, and it occurred to me that perhaps she didn't mean it so philosophically. Perhaps she only meant this: that we have to learn our hard edges, the outlines of ourselves, the habits and minute pleasures that give us weight in the world, the lines we will not cross, the lines we will, the shape not of our lives as a whole – who, after all, can ever know what comes next? – but of our lives in miniature, on a day-to-day basis. And perhaps I have only just begun to do this.

4

What Remains

The pregnancy goes well until it doesn't. One week, then another, then another. Technically I am allowed to swim now, but I can't quite bring myself to start going to the pool again. I think, I'll just wait another week. I'll wait until I've met the midwife. Eventually I think: well, I've waited this long, I'll wait until the twelve-week scan, the end of the first trimester. A part of me is always on edge, but another part of me, as time goes by, begins to be open to the possibility that everything might be OK.

And then one evening, a few days shy of the twelve-week milestone, the point at which many people choose to announce a pregnancy, preferring to wait until the likelihood of miscarriage has dropped, I begin to bleed. It is heavy. And yet the next day when we arrive at the Early Pregnancy Assessment Unit expecting the worst there instead is an image so like all those scans I'd seen posted to Facebook or Instagram, an image of a *baby*, or the beginnings of one, so much more palpable and recognisable than we'd expected: limbs, belly, a button nose – and there, crucially, the beating heart.

At first it seems like that was it; the bleeding eases off, we breathe easy over the weekend. On Monday I have an appointment with my acupuncturist and she tells me about another client of hers who'd had a similar experience, had bled for weeks and found it intensely stressful, but who had in the end given birth to a perfectly healthy baby. But the next morning I wake up feeling ill, feverish; I begin to panic, call my GP, who sees me that afternoon and says it is impossible to tell: the two things might be connected, but the more likely explanation is coincidence – I have a virus, the timing is just bad. Coincidence or not, that evening I begin to bleed even more heavily, so heavily that it seems impossible anything could survive or remain. The EPAU sees me the next day, at twelve weeks exactly, and there again is that image, there again is that reassuring heartbeat. I am still bleeding, but my official twelve-week scan, which can be done anytime between ten and fourteen weeks, is on Saturday; I will not have to wait too long for another glimpse, more reassurance. With the proviso that I call if anything changes they release me into the world and we feel cautiously giddy. I have arranged for someone to cover my lectures for the week and Alexander can't concentrate on work, so we decide to drive to Aylesbury to look at a car we are interested in buying to replace our twenty-year-old Yaris, which has a habit of breaking down at inconvenient moments and which will, we've been told, definitely fail its next MOT.

As we drive the bleeding intensifies. I bleed through my leggings, onto the seat of the car, and we stop at a Tesco superstore on the outskirts of Aylesbury so that I can buy new pants, new leggings, a fresh pack of high-absorbency pads. When we get in the new car for a test drive I am worried about bleeding onto the seat, so I keep my coat on even though it is boiling inside and cross my legs tightly, as if I can will the bleeding to ease off. The day is bright, late March, the edge of spring, a softness in the air. I see us as an outsider might: a young couple, expecting their first baby, in the market for a safer, more serious car, thinking about the future.

The car is smooth and quiet. We have not looked at any others but impulsively we agree to come back at the weekend to pay for it and go through the paperwork. We drive home. I lie on the couch, still bleeding, but resolutely detached: who knows what is going on, who knows what the outcome will be, my acupuncturist had a client . . .

From the parking lot of the Tesco I had called a colleague at the university who was covering my teaching to explain why I couldn't come in again on Friday. I didn't need to explain, I didn't feel obliged, except that it seemed to me that I owed her honesty, and she'd repaid me in kind: I've been through that too, she'd said, just look after yourself, and a weight was briefly lifted from my shoulders, in spite of the circumstances.

For two days I move about the house like a ghost, going from couch to couch, watching endless episodes of *Outlander*, proof-reading an epic historical romance for a publisher, monitoring the bleeding. On Friday an old friend comes round for a cup of tea; we sit in the living room, and she tells me that she'd bled when she'd been pregnant with her son. Even though I know her experience does not necessarily have any bearing on mine it is soothing nonetheless to hear her speak in retrospect, soothing just to hear her speak, as if I am still a part of the world.

On Saturday we drive to the hospital for the long-awaited twelve-week scan. We arrive on a floor of the maternity ward that I have never been to: we have never got this far into the journey before. My heart is thumping in my chest. The receptionist tells us they are running behind schedule and they will get to us when they get to us. We sit in a waiting area. Most of the other women are visibly pregnant, leaning back in their seats, rubbing protruding bellies. On a TV screen a series of informational animations and advertisements runs on a loop: a whole new set of things to worry about. Is your baby kicking regularly? Or: Help reduce the risk of SIDS! Next to me a young woman, she looks like she is in her early twenties at the oldest, sits jiggling her leg. On one side of her is a young man, perhaps the baby's father, and on the other a middle-aged woman, perhaps her mother or mother-in-law, and she is saying to one or both of them, pointing at her belly, 'well, when this baby comes . . .', and I think about the luxury of that *when*, the optimism of it. I have begun to experience a gentle cramping, I have no right or no courage to say *when*. Across from us a machine dishes out ultrasound images, £5 each. When the nurse comes to collect us she looks exhausted, frustrated. She leads us into the room and introduces us to another woman, who is not in uniform. I'm not really an ultrasound technician, she begins, then shakes her head, tries again: I mean, I am, but not *here*. I'm interviewing for a job. I'll be doing your scan, if that's OK. She doesn't say it as a question. They are on a tight schedule and I have to fight to squeeze my words in, to tell them about the bleeding, about the other scans. I can't tell if they are interested or annoyed – I feel, but I may be projecting, that their job is only with the *healthy* pregnancies, they deal in joy and instructions on how to operate the £5-a-photo machine, they do not need this complication today, but they duly squeeze the gel onto my stomach, go about their business.

I can see that something isn't right, I have learned to spot that flash of the heartbeat and before they say anything I know it isn't there. The nurses seem embarrassed. They leave the room briefly, to give us time to collect ourselves, although we are already pretty well collected, in my opinion: we have become good at absorbing bad news in these intimate, compromising positions. I wipe the gel from my belly and bury my head briefly in Alexander's chest. Then the nurse who works for the hospital leads us away, bypassing the waiting room full of pregnant women, down corridors and stairwells, until we arrive in the area of the hospital we *are* familiar with, know well, the area where they deal with the things that go wrong. She leaves us sitting in another waiting room and disappears through a set of doors, comes back a few minutes later to say it will be at least an hour or two before a doctor can see us, we may as well go and get a coffee and come back, and leaves us there with visible relief. The relief is not unkind, in fact it is perfectly understandable; this is not the outcome she would have wanted for us either, I'm sure, and if I could leave the frustration of it, the sadness, down in this basement room right now and take the elevator back up to a place with happier outcomes I would do it too.

We have our coffee outside on a patio somewhere in the maze of the hospital complex. It is weak, bitter. There are other people sitting outside too, some of them obviously sick, attached to IV drips or with recently stitched wounds visible. We sit saying very little; I don't know about Alexander but I feel that if I say too much I might begin to cry, and it seems obscene somehow to cry here; on this hospital patio, in this unseasonable warmth, it seems insensitive. Then, because we still have time to kill, we go for a walk. At the top of the hill is a small park, and the sun is shining, and we walk the perimeter of the park, watching small children toddle happily. I think, or maybe I say out loud: *we'll have our own toddler someday too.* Not because I necessarily believe it, but because it seems that there can be no way to start to believe it without first articulating it.

The doctor, when she finally sees us, can tell us nothing we don't already know. Because it is the weekend they can't schedule me for a D&C, if that's what I want, but I can call on Monday to make arrangements. In the meantime, if I do pass the products of conception, I can, if I want, save them and bring them in for analysis.

What can we do? It is early afternoon. We call our parents, to tell them the news. We call a few friends who we had told about the IVF, the pregnancy, the bleeding. We go and collect our new car, as we'd promised the salesman we would; Alexander's father drives us there, we listen to Radio 4 on the way and speak only intermittently. We meet friends for a drink at the pub; I have a large glass of red wine and talk fast, flushed and flustered, almost giddy. The wine relaxes me, fuzzes my thoughts, but the light hangs on late and we sleep restlessly.

The next day – Mothering Sunday, as it happens, a detail that in a novel or a film might feel overwrought – the cramping, which before had been merely an undercurrent, intensifies until I think, irrationally, that perhaps I can't endure it. I call the hospital and they suggest a hot water bottle. When I go to the loo I bleed, and then I feel the drop of the amniotic sac. I catch it in a bed of loo roll and deposit it into a Tupperware that Alexander brings up from the kitchen. I call the hospital again and they recommend we put it in the fridge, if we can bear to, until we can bring it in for analysis.

Perhaps it's terrible to say, but the physical relief is immediate and overpowering: suddenly I feel not a twinge, not a whisper of pain, in fact I feel light and powerful. In the early evening we go out to our old car and clear it of all our belongings, so that Alexander can take it to our local branch of We Buy Any Car. I scrub half-heartedly at the small spot of blood on the passenger seat for a moment, then give up.

When we see the doctor on Monday we hand over the Tupperware, and we all laugh about it. How can we not? What else is there to do? She says it looks and sounds as if I have passed everything, that the bleeding should resolve in a few weeks, that I should take a pregnancy test in three weeks to confirm, that otherwise – the usual saying – I should *proceed as normal*.

Well, what is normal? But it's not as hard as it sounds: another warm spring day, a drive into town, a soda and a sandwich for lunch. Buy something frivolous, a cushion cover or a pretty ceramic plant pot. At home, as dusk starts to darken the rooms, turn the lights on, email your students to tell them their lecture will be held at the usual time this week, cook dinner, lie on the couch together watching a film you'll later forget, go to bed later than you meant to. Wake up and do it again, or something like it.

*

Still: the frustration of it, the nearness, the almost-thereness. The dearness of that image, the clearness: who could help but get attached at that point, even if they knew better than to assume? The sadness of it, which continues for a while to hit at strange moments, and not so strange ones. Reading a version of *The Epic of Gilgamesh* as recounted in Robert Macfarlane's *Underland*: Gilgamesh's servant Enki returning from the realm of the dead, the 'netherworld', where he has journeyed to try to retrieve a lost object. *'Did you see my little stillborn children who never knew existence?'* asks Gilgamesh. *'I saw them,'* answers Enki. Or, in that same book, a reference to what Elaine Scarry has called the *deep subterranean fact* of pain; Scarry was writing of physical pain specifically, but it also seems as good a way as any I have found to describe the particular pain of this kind of loss, a deep thing, under the surface, hidden, kept. I would not say that these things unravel or unsettle me so much as strike me, in a kind of violent way; my head snaps back, the blood hums in my ears, I think, *oh*.

The night Notre-Dame burns I find myself in floods of tears. It means nothing to me, I have been there only once, over a decade ago, my first summer in the UK, when I had gone to Paris by myself for a weekend. I had stayed in a shabby hotel on a busy road near the Place de la République, splurging on a €50-a-night en suite. I spoke no French, knew no one in the city, had only a flimsy guidebook I had picked up at the Gare du Nord on arrival and no real agenda, and so for two days all I did was walk. I walked everywhere, miles and miles, in loops, from the Louvre to the Latin Quarter to the Eiffel Tower to the Sacré-Cœur to the Grande Mosquée, where I nursed a mint tea that reminded me of being in Fez with Alexander earlier in the summer. On one of my walks I came to Notre-Dame and I went inside and was surprised by how crowded it was, and how big. On a disposable camera, because, drunk, I had lost my digital camera earlier in the summer, I took some very poor photographs of the stained-glass windows, the high ceilings. I went across the river and had a coffee. I had only met Alexander two months ago, but I missed him, I wished he was with me. I sent him a text message, I went on walking. I was twenty years old, anything might happen, but already I felt the future narrowing, or solidifying: a few months ago I would have relished the freedom to go out in a new city and meet new people, but now what I wanted was much more insular, I wanted the comfort of a relationship, I wanted the person I was in a couple with to be sitting on the other side of the table, and no one else. After this summer I had a semester left of university and then who knew – except that I was starting to know, I was starting in my heart but also in my head to make a commitment.

Now, almost twelve years later, the cathedral up in flames, Twitter alight with videos and commentary, I read a quote from a cathedral spokesperson and feel it like a punch in the gut: *everything is burning, nothing will remain from the frame.* Stupid, of course: it is sad that the cathedral is burning, but I know deep down that isn't why *I* am sad, or at least, that isn't why I am *so* sad. Or maybe it is, in a roundabout way, but either way it is a selfish sadness, at its core.

*

But this time we know. What is it we know? We know that it gets easier. We know that we will be OK, one way or another. We know that we have things to look forward to, in the immediate future, though probably in the deeper future, too. We know that we still have four more embryos in the freezer and an appointment scheduled with a recurrent miscarriage specialist. We know each other well enough to speak freely, to laugh about things that deserve to be laughed about, to make plans, to have a few pints on a weekend evening, to drink our coffee outside, to plant new things out, foxgloves, radishes. We know that the seasons are changing, the days are getting longer, the tulips and the plum blossom have erupted in the garden. We know that after all something remains from the frame.

5
Tiger

That spring is a riot of birdsong and bloom. The streets all smell sweet with rain and honeysuckle and the light hangs on hopefully, much past its winter bedtime, and whenever I go outside and stand in the garden there are birds, birds, birds – the keen of a red kite, the whistle of a pigeon, a hundred other chirps and chimes that I can't identify, but in concert they even seem to outweigh the persistent hum of the traffic.

In that time I write our landlady an email to ask if we can make some updates to the kitchen. In the email I explain our circumstances, I say that I have just been through a cycle of IVF that ended in a miscarriage, that we will probably do another before too long, that we are therefore keen to get the work done sooner than later. I am struck by both her kindness and her sagacity in response. *Do enjoy the spring,* she writes at the end of the email. *That can help with everything.* And it does.

(Every time I have done this, every time I have disclosed a truth like this – to a colleague, a landlady, even a friend or an acquaintance – I have felt I've risked something. I can afford to, of course: my privilege, my position, make the stakes low enough. If I lose my job, for example, well, it would be awful, it would be hard, but it would not be *the end*; if I alienate someone by sharing too much, if I embarrass them, or myself, I will be all right. Still: every time I am glad I have done it. I have met more kindness, more empathy, than I had known possible.)

★

Perhaps it is time to return to the water. To the feel of it, the flow of it. To the pool. I have strayed away from it, both in my habits and in my mind. Perhaps it has come to represent something of myself that I do not recognise any more, or something that I am struggling to regain. I thought it would help me make sense of my situation, but that was before I knew that I don't know, might never know, what my situation actually *is*. There will in all likelihood never be a definitive answer, no conclusion: no one will ever say to us *this* is why things went wrong, *this* is what you can do to fix it. There is no diagnosis, there is no reason, or not one that anyone can perceive, anyhow. There is only what will be, or what won't be.

When Alexander and I first decided that *now* was the time that we wanted to make and have a baby, we did not really understand what *now* is. There was so much we did not understand — so much in the abstract, about resilience, about balance, about how to be kind to each other, but also, more banally, about the actual logistics of conception, the sheer unlikelihood of it, really, all the ways it might go wrong — but particularly we did not know this: that *now* has happened, is happening, will happen, no matter what plan has or has not materialised. We did not understand the fluidity and the tenderness of everything, the way time slips and flows away from us, the way our own time is precious even when we spend it on nothing in particular.

In a way the pool has in fact helped me make sense of it. I remember that at the start of his wild swimming opus, *Waterlog*, Roger Deakin compares the swimming pool to a cage. Breaststroking up and down the length of the moat at his house in Suffolk while a summer downpour pocks the water around him, Deakin resolves to embark on a journey through the open waters of Britain — streams, rivers, lakes, ponds. *I wanted to follow the rain on its meanderings about our land to rejoin the sea,* he writes, *to break out of the frustration of a lifetime doing lengths, of endlessly turning back on myself like a tiger pacing its cage.*

Am I the tiger? Is the pool a cage? Have I been a captive all this time – by the walls, the ceiling, the rigidity of habit and compulsion, by the narrow-mindedness of obsession?

I think of it: the rectangle, the straight lines, the circular sweep of the hands on the clocks that hang on the wall, one at each end of the pool, the tick tock beating steadily against the linear backdrop of the lanes. The back and forth. But then again perhaps it's not the pool itself that is the cage, but merely my dependence on it. Perhaps the problem has been in thinking that understanding a problem or a desire or a preoccupation is the only solution, the only justification, the only way to move forward.

And how can I write about the passage of time, about the clocks on the wall, without returning to this: the empty room, the heartbeat seen or not seen, the biological clock?

Tick tock, tick tock, it says still, even now. Another kind of cage, another kind of trap.

My only response, for so long, has been to repeat myself. I have chosen the same locker, the same lane. I have put my cap on in front of the mirror in the changing room and thought a hopeful little mantra to myself. I have rinsed my goggles in the shower before pressing them around my eyes. I have stood at the edge, so many times, for a few moments longer than necessary, stretching my arms or pretending to fuss with the straps of my goggles, delaying the shock of immersion. I have let phrases drift through my head as I swim, the same few words, over and over again. Superstitions, really: rituals that can't, I know, but somehow must, I feel, influence other parts of my life. I have thought that if I do everything exactly right, in exactly the right order, then the universe will have no choice but to bend to my will.

But maybe it's just that sameness is soothing, sometimes: it tells us that we're still us, we're still here, we're still OK. Maybe I shouldn't read any more into it than that.

★

One Monday morning in early May, a bank holiday, I sit outside after my first swim in five months. The temperature is so perfect that it feels like the air is part of me, or I it, and it is so quiet: no traffic, no shouts, no music. I want to hold on to that feeling, that sweetness, Alexander still asleep upstairs, the muted sounds of the neighbours at home, the house cooler than the air outside, so that to step out is to be wrapped round, held loosely but safely, in a warmth.

For my first swim I chose not to go to my usual pool but to the lido on the other side of town. I had not seen anyone I knew. I had not counted lengths. I had not said to myself beforehand: you must do at least twenty laps, or stay in for at least half an hour; I did not even wear a watch. It was just me and the water, a little mist rising from the surface. Afterwards I'd cycled home along the river path, bending around runners and dog walkers. I had not had any particular compulsion that morning to go to the indoor pool, to *my* pool. I have been away for so long, in fact, that it no longer seems to belong to me at all. How can I explain my absence? Will I need to? Will things have changed beyond recognition?

Sitting there in the garden in the stillness, the silence, I feel something like a loosening, a freeing in my chest. For so many years I have held myself hostage to the necessity of routine, to the rigid lines of superstitious repetition. I have been compelled, held. Once, years ago, I remember thinking that I wasn't sure I could consider moving anywhere – back home to the ranch where I grew up, for example – where I couldn't be within walking distance of a pool. But what if my own obsession has been trapping me? What if it was just a helpful metaphor that has now outlived its usefulness? What if I never return to that particular way of being? What if that is no bad thing?

A week or so later, a Sunday, I rise early and cycle to the pool, my pool, just like old times. The streets are warm and empty. The pool is warm and empty. Everything is familiar but not familiar. In the changing room I hesitate at a locker, struggling with the lock, in a reverie which is broken eventually by a woman standing beside me – here, she says, you need to turn the dial like this. Oh, I laugh, I know. I've been coming here for years, I say, more to convince myself than her, I was just having one of those moments. Zoned out. Somewhere else. She laughs too. We certainly all have those! she says. Then adds: I just wondered if maybe you were new here. *Well, maybe I am, in a way*, I think.

After my swim I cycle home and make a pot of coffee and drink it in the garden, swaddled under a large jumper, listening to the neighbours' kids in their garden, observing the wild-flowers bending in a subtle wind. I feel good, better certainly than I would had I stayed inside, in bed, but I also don't feel as if anything is riding on it, like I will dissolve if I don't keep showing up, like it is part of the theatre of control.

Will I go again tomorrow? I ask myself.

Maybe, maybe not, I think. I don't have to decide now.

6

A Luxury

Oh, I know: this is a luxury, all of it. The wishing, the wondering, the waiting, the hoping, but also the despair, the anger, the sadness, the anxiety. The IVF, of course. The pregnancy tests, the ovulation tests – £15 to pee on a stick and throw it away! – the vitamins, the non-alcoholic beers, the fresh spinach, the fish, the salads, the beetroot from our garden, pickled in a jar, the *time*, the sheer amount of time. The time we've wasted, the time we've spent, the time we still have. *You're still young*, and it's true, I am, even now. Even the decision itself, and every subsequent decision, is a luxury, a luxury that not everyone – not even most people – has. Let us not forget that. Let us not forget, either, that this is a fact, not necessarily a consolation.

7

Ours

About a year before our first round of IVF, I went to dinner
with some friends. There were seven of us in a cramped upstairs
restaurant in East London, three couples and me, Alexander
being otherwise engaged. It was good, the restaurant, the company. I was having fun, I even caught myself, reapplying lipstick
in the bathroom, thinking of how happy I was, in that moment,
with my situation. With my friends. With the food and the wine
and the exhibit we'd been to at the museum earlier. I'd finally
got my PhD, I had some lecturing work lined up, I was wearing
new boots, I felt like a grown-up. Maybe I was, in that moment,
even a little glad that Alexander wasn't there, even though
everyone had asked after him, even though it would have been
nice to lean into him at the cramped table, because it gave me
a chance to be whoever I felt I was in that moment without his
intervention, or without my intervention into his own way of
being – the constant social negotiation of marriage, each person
trying to be both who they are as a couple and, at the same time,
who they are as an individual.

And then – still in this moment – I was hit with another
thought: that maybe, probably, in all likelihood, this was the last
time we would all be together like this. One couple had a new
puppy; they were taking turns to go anxiously but excitedly
to the window, through which they could see the pup in their
car, every ten minutes or so. Soon enough, though, it would be
a baby, surely. We were all in our thirties: how long until this

kind of late-night gathering would become unthinkable? How unlikely it was that we would all be in exactly the same place for much longer. How natural, and yet somehow alarming to ponder, that soon – *tick, tock* – we would disperse, that soon some of us would be subsumed by parenthood and its attendant worries and responsibilities, that others, whether by choice or by necessity or by a little of both, would not.

I of course had already started down the next road, and had already got stuck. I had some insight into what awaited some of us, the unlucky, the badly built. I knew there was always the possibility of struggle, of that explosive meeting of desire and inability. I also knew that assuming everyone at that table wanted to have their own children, they probably would. There were four women: statistically only one of us would miscarry; maybe I was just the statistic – but of course statistics are not that simple, and I knew for a fact, anyhow, that at least two of us already had. I knew deep down, too, that it was not just about the maths; that *want* is complicated, that relationships are, bodies are, that decisions are, that friendships are. But for a moment what I knew was eclipsed by what I felt, which was a quick thrum of fear: *they would all leave us behind.*

I came back to the table a little sobered. I sipped my wine and tried to evaluate the feeling. What difference did it make, really, if or when other people had children? It was not a competition – but of course a part of me could not let go of the idea that it was, that somehow, if I failed to reproduce, it would be just that, a *failure*, that I would be stuck, that everyone else would move on with their lives, move forwards, and I would be forever *here*, losing the race. What was it I feared most in that moment? That Alexander and I would never be parents, or that, if we weren't, all these people, with their normal middle-class lives, their career-marriage-house-baby trajectories, would pity us? That we would pity ourselves?

★

Later I would read a passage in Sheila Heti's *Motherhood*, in which Heti talks about what the choice not to have children looks like to those who have chosen to have them. *I fear that without children,* she writes, *it doesn't look like you have made a choice, or that you're doing anything but just continuing on – drifting. People who don't have children might be thought not to move forward, or change and grow, or have stories that build on stories, or lives of ever-increasing depth and love and pain. Maybe they seem stalled in one place – a place the parents have left behind.* And even though she's writing about *choice*, and not about the murky area where choice cannot necessarily account for what does or does not happen, I felt keenly the truth of what she was saying: that having children, not having them, are not hierarchical states of being. And who was I to view anyone's life – even, or especially, my own – as if it was stuck, undeveloped, simply because it had a different shape to the one I had imagined it should take? My husband and I didn't have children yet, it was true, and maybe we never would, but, I saw, we were not simply stalled in the place the parents had already left behind, we were somewhere new, somewhere our own, we had lives of *ever-increasing depth and love and pain.*

Shouldn't that have been obvious from the outset? But it wasn't.

*

I think sometimes about what it means that Alexander and I are in this together. I think about the things I have said in anger and in fear, the ways I have tried to punish myself by pushing him away, the selfishness of my outbursts, of my suggestions that he feel free to leave, to find someone else, to *get on with your life,* the image I have had of him with another woman, holding their child.

I am not sentimental about this; I have never believed, and he has never believed either, that there is only one person with whom you can happily go through life. If we had not met each other we each would have found someone else, someone else with whom we could be equally happy, happier maybe, in some ways. But we did meet each other, and there's no going back from that. Yes, I have said, and thought, terrible things, and maybe even meant them, in the heat of the moment. *Find someone else, another woman, one of those hyper-fertile ones, who seem to fall pregnant if you breathe on them the right way.*

But he could not – and neither could I – countenance that. It would be like giving up some essential part of yourself, losing a limb. And somehow every time something has gone wrong, every time something has been difficult, it has felt like a kind of drawing closer, not apart. *Get on with your life*: but this is his life, and mine. It is ours. We made it, keep making it.

8

A Record

The arbitrariness of endings: all stories are circles, in a way, and in that way they are restrictive, reductive – *like a diagnosis*, the novelist Sarah Moss writes, *a story can become a prison*. When I think about the narratives I know about fertility, the narratives that are told, they seem so well defined, so black and white, so neatly packaged, even the ones that are messy. Stories like: they waited years. And years. And years again. And then they gave up. And then – biblically – a child was born unto them. Or: they waited and nothing. Full stop. But they found meaning elsewhere. Consolation. Peace. A sense of purpose.

But what if you are still in limbo, still unsure of what you want or what you'll get? If I have learned anything from all these years of waiting, wondering, not-knowing, it is this: that there is always someone else adrift. You are not the only one. The voices carried through paper-thin curtains separating each woman and her pain from the next; the knowing glances in waiting rooms; the sudden, casual revelation at a pub table: *oh, we're going through that too*. Our lives only look neat in retrospect; most of the time we're just muddling through.

For so long, I was afraid of what it would mean to say any of this out loud. I was silent, because it felt to me that until there was a story, an ending, I had no right to speak. But the silence is too much. I can't not speak, even if there's nothing conclusive to say – no, precisely *because* there's nothing conclusive to say.

To write this, then, is an act of faith. Not long ago I realised that after my first miscarriage I wrote one essay – a small thing, published online, at a now-defunct website – and then nothing, not for years. I published nothing else, I hardly even wrote in my notebook, I who had always taken meticulous notes about everything, I who had identified first and foremost as a *writer* for so long. I had to start saying to people who thought I was, who asked where I was writing, or what: oh no, I'm not really a writer, I haven't written anything for years!

I grasped a silence, and then I held so tight to it that it became a part of me.

I thought that I had to wait for an outcome. I thought that in the meantime if I wrote it, any of it, I would be tempting fate. Or that I would misspeak, misrepresent somehow my own experience, my own grief or anxiety, and that people would be upset, or offended, or alienated, when what I wanted was the opposite – to feel closer to others, with their grief and anxiety, to create a sense of shared experience. Or I thought that they would simply say: shut up. Suck it up. Move on. And I would not be able to explain: that's exactly what I want, too. That's exactly what I'm trying to do. Don't you see?

I gave myself to the silence. I lost years over it. Lost is an exaggeration, of course, it's melodramatic. But for as long as the obsession was only felt, and not articulated, I think I ceased to be myself. I worried, speaking to that acupuncturist, about whether I would be able to give up enough, when really I had already given up too much.

I have little to show for all this time: like the trace of a hand through water, there's a ripple and then nothing. But what if you give that time, that silence, a shape? If you do that, then it becomes something.

If we do have a child, I wonder, will these words cease to mean anything? Will I want them to disappear? Will all this matter less, or not at all? It will, in a way, I know: suddenly we will be starting fresh, suddenly the years of worry and waiting will seem like nothing, will seem like a waste, perhaps we should just have sat back and relaxed and let it come in its own time, perhaps this, perhaps that. If we don't, too, will it someday seem as if we should not have spent so long here, in this place, when we could have just been getting on with something else?

But that is exactly why to write the words down, exactly why to record what it feels like here, because it is a vanishing place, and if, when, it vanishes for us, nothing will be left of it but the trace, the memory, the imperfect picture I've sketched here, the ripple in the water.

So I want a record, something inscribed in stone – sunk *deeply into an unchanging place* – I want something that says, like the carving in the tree, *we were here.* I don't want to forget a thing, a place, that marked me, or made me. I don't want to diminish it, or belittle it, or pretend it didn't, or pretend it meant nothing, in the end. That would be to do it, and myself, and everyone else who is here, has been here, will be here, a great disservice.

So there is no resolution, I'm sorry – but also not sorry – to say. I'm going to keep going up and down the length of the pool, when I can – because I don't know what else to do, but also because it's a thing I can count on. I consider myself lucky that I can show up on a Tuesday morning in September, say, and go through familiar motions, and smile hello to women whose swimming strokes and habits I know so well. Even after all these years I know little else about them – a name here and there, an occupation, with one woman sometimes I go to a café nearby after our swim and we have coffee and cinnamon buns and chat about our work, which is similar, but I don't need to pry, to know more. It is enough that I am recognised. That I recognise. That's it. I have, let's say, another decade, maybe more, of drunken conversations in pubs, of not knowing, of silently recognising, of wishing, of agreeing that yes, it's still possible, yes, I'm still more or less young, before anyone will look at me and wonder what happened, why not. Or, alternatively, will look at me and not have to wonder at all, and not know what it took to get there. And in the meantime I will make this place, wherever it is, as much my home as I can.

9

Listen I Love You

A bright Saturday afternoon in October. It is 2019: more than six years now since that first definitive conversation by the river, the decision, the timelines in the notebook, the abandoned pack of pills. Six years since we first set tentative foot in this place, since I entered this ambiguous realm of almost, maybe.

I am sitting on the couch. Sunlight is coming through the bay window, a cobweb is clinging to the sill, shivering in a draught. On the mantelpiece a late-season rose in a vase has opened like the dawn, filling the room with its scent and peachy warmth.

I should be giving birth today, or one of these days: another missed due date. Instead we are in the midst of our second cycle of IVF.

Perhaps I ought to be sadder about this, to feel the failure of it, the *should*, more keenly. There in the hallway the ghost of a hospital bag, there in the room upstairs the ghost of a cot, which we would surely have bought by now, there in front of me the ghost of a belly grown to its fullest extent, fit to burst.

But the simple fact is it is also nice just to be sitting here on the couch in the sunlight, reading, waiting.

Yesterday in the rain we drove up the road to the fertility clinic for the embryo transfer. We arrived early and walked once round the parking lot before going in, to kill some time. There was no one else in the waiting room. Through a plexiglass window we could see into the lab, where people in scrubs and hairnets moved about. One of them on a mobile phone, throwing her head back and laughing. Were they all there for us? Of course not: but for a moment it felt that way, this whole army of embryologists there only to serve us, our whim, our will. *Good luck!* everyone we saw in the clinic said to us, as if luck has anything to do with it – or perhaps luck has everything to do with it.

In the treatment room I lay back on the bed and put my feet in the stirrups, a blue plastic sheet draped over my legs, and repeated my name and my date of birth. A doctor and a nurse, and in a doorway to the lab an embryologist holding a small petri dish. All women. The nurse squeezed gel onto my stomach and operated the probe so that the doctor would have a clear picture of my uterus. The doctor received the embryo and inserted the catheter. Alexander held my hand. The doctor removed the catheter and we all looked at the screen.

Can you see it? A bright spot, the doctor said, and there it was.

Later at home I thought of the opening lines to Julia Copus's poem 'Pledge': *Chiel, adrift / in the deeps of the future, / twiripe, yet-to-be / son or daughter.*

Who knows what will come of it, who knows what the deeps of the future hold.

Last week my therapist, a new one, said in reference to my situation: *it's as if you're swimming in a pool, trying to get from one end to the other.* It was uncanny: for a moment I couldn't speak. *I don't know if that makes sense*, she said, perhaps thinking that I did not understand, but I was only amazed: had I talked to her at all about swimming pools? No, I was sure I hadn't, though I had mentioned once or twice that I liked to swim, for exercise. She had no reason to alight on that phrase in particular, and yet there it was.

Yes, I said. It makes sense.

★

My grandmother has stopped swimming. She is ninety-five. It makes her too tired, she says, she doesn't have the energy for it, although in other ways she is still extremely active. She still patrols the parcel of land on which she and my parents live, tending the rose bushes, the orange trees, the macadamia orchard, which she planted more than thirty years ago, carefully propagating varieties based on instinct and the advice of an eccentric expert. She is a ruthless gardener: if something shows weakness she rips it out without a second thought, without any sentimentality. My father has offered to drive her to the pool, and then straight back to the house, so that she can get in the water for even just a few minutes, but she has declined, drawn a line under it, unsentimental as always: fifty years of swimming isn't bad going, she said. So that's that.

For years she and I have kept up a regular correspondence via email, and for most of those years our primary subject was swimming. We exchanged updates about conditions at our respective pools, and about our strokes and our fitness. We addressed little else; this was what we had in common, a shared language, not secret, exactly, but coded somehow.

Me: *The temperature here is just above freezing and all the trees are bare. It's nice to swim indoors in winter, when it's too cold and dark to stay outside for very long.*

Her: *Today the sky was full of interesting clouds and birds, the water was warm and the pool was empty except for one other swimmer, and I still remembered how to swim.*

Because I live far away from where I grew up, I sometimes find it hard to trace myself, to see where exactly it is that I am rooted to this earth, but then I remember that some of it, a large part of it, is there, in those emails. There's an irrefutability to them, and so to me. I swim because I can, and because it's a form of continuity, but it isn't the only thing that links me to the world.

For a time, when I learned that my grandmother had stopped swimming, I thought: *now what will we write about?* But there is so much: the weather, the rain, the drought, the garden, the roses, the fruit trees.

I myself, meanwhile, have not been for a swim in over a month. Do I miss it? The honest answer is: yes and no. Before we started this cycle, when summer was still clinging on, I was going to the pool quite regularly, though not as frequently as I used to – three mornings a week, maybe. It felt like a gift, not a necessity. I knew that I'd have to stop soon. It was a quiet time of year, many people away for the summer, the students dispersed, and very often I would have a lane to myself, or else I would share with one of the other regulars; we had made an agreement that even though our speeds differed we preferred to swim with people we knew, whose behaviour we could predict, who we could pause and chat to when we grew tired. Yes: that's a nice feeling, and so is immersion itself, and very often these days I have dreams which are an expression of yearning to be in water. I dream that I am at home, on the ranch, and my visit is coming to an end and I still have not been in the ocean, and it's getting dark, or I have something else to do; I dream that the water level in the pool is so low that I am not swimming but crawling along the bottom; once, gloriously, I dream that we are at the seaside and I have no costume, but I fling myself in anyhow, in my pants and bra. But it seems to me that I have been going to the pool for long enough now that either way, no matter what happens, the next time I visit, whether it's in a few weeks or a few months, it will still feel like a form of home – and so too, I hope, I think, I'm almost certain, will my body, whether I'm pregnant or not.

*

So yes, here is where we are: it could go either way. The two-week wait, which is not actually quite two weeks but twelve days. At the end of the wait you wake up and take a pregnancy test. But of course no matter what the result of the test is there are still a thousand what ifs, a thousand maybes, a thousand worries, a thousand possibilities, a thousand things that could happen.

There's a walk I've taken to doing, in the mornings, before work, instead of a swim, through a nature reserve near our house. As I walk sometimes I make in my head a list of things that give me pleasure. Sunlight on grass. A swim in the ocean, followed by a warm jumper and a cold beer. A cup of coffee and a good book on a Saturday morning. Seeing the house lit up from the inside, knowing Alexander is home, cooking dinner. It's not that I think I can transcend grander ambitions by focusing only on small satisfactions. It's not that I'm not aware of discomforts or anxieties or insecurities. I have a lot of questions about the bigger picture. Are we really any better equipped to bring a child into this world than we were six years ago? We have a more stable income, true, and I am no longer a PhD student, but we still have precious little in the way of savings or security, we still do not own a home, we still do not hoover frequently enough, or floss, and meanwhile every day on the news is more evidence of widespread societal precarity. The world, I know, will not get any easier to live in. It will ask questions of us that we will not be able to answer. Are we a burden on the NHS? What about global poverty, the threat of pandemic, the vastness of the climate crisis? Is it irresponsible in the face of all this to want, to hope? Or is it the only thing, under the circumstances, we can do?

But on these walks, enjoying for example the sunlight on my face, there's always a moment where it's possible to hold many potential outcomes, many potential answers, at once, and still feel solid, and reassured.

★

The poem that found me, the day before the embryo transfer, was Kim Addonizio's 'To the Woman Crying Uncontrollably in the Next Stall', and its explosive last line:

listen I love you joy is coming

Lying in bed I read that and I felt with a rare conviction that one way or another I believe it's true. I believe it's true whatever happens at the end of this two-week wait, whatever happens after that, whatever path we find ourselves on. And if that's the only good thing to come out of all this – but I know it isn't – it's enough. It's enough.

Acknowledgements

From the beginning, I've been fortunate to have had in Harriet Moore the most perceptive and patient agent I could possibly have hoped for. This book certainly would never have come into being, let alone found its home, without her. That home, the perfect home, was with Jenny Lord at W&N, and I am similarly indebted to Jenny for her clarity of vision and her smart, sensitive feedback. She saw what this book was even before I did, and guided it there with great editorial skill.

Many thanks also to Sarah Fortune, Kate Moreton and Virginia Woolstencroft at W&N for all their brilliant work, to Steve Marking for the beautiful cover design, to Martha Sprackland for her astute copyedit, and to Clare Hubbard for her proofreading skill.

In 2019 I was lucky enough to receive an Authors' Foundation grant from the Society of Authors, which proved instrumental in allowing me some time and space to work on *Adrift*. Much gratitude to the SoA for their commitment to offering financial assistance to writers for works in progress.

This book has origins in the research I conducted as part of my PhD at Royal Holloway, University of London. I am grateful to many members of the geography department there, past and present, for their encouragement and intellectual generosity, but to Phil Crang in particular for his support, especially throughout some of the events described in these pages.

Thanks to Elizabeth Garner and Joanna Walsh for conversations and reassurance about the process of writing (and selling) a book. Sophie Ratcliffe has been friend, mentor, cheerleader and an utter inspiration to me, and I will be forever grateful to have her in my life. And I owe a great deal both personally and professionally to John Mitchinson and Rachael Kerr, whose friendship is very dear.

In these pages I have often featured conversations with friends and family, borrowing their anecdotes to serve my own purpose. I'm grateful for the openness of everyone whose stories feature here, in whatever way, and I hope I have represented their experiences with emotional, if not always literal, veracity. To a great extent, though, a memoir is an exercise in (mis)remembering, always from the limited point of view of I – and so any inaccuracies here are mine and mine alone.

In writing about the medical events described in this book I have similarly relied primarily upon my own fallible memory, as well as notes taken at emotionally vulnerable moments. If in my ignorance I have made any mistakes, blame no one but the unreliable narrator that is my body.

On the subject of medicine: I have been fortunate throughout the events described in this book – and beyond – to have received wonderful care and compassion from doctors, nurses, midwives, counsellors and many others. To someone born in a country whose default approach to healthcare provision has historically been frankly inhumane, the ease with which I was able to access this care was astonishing. I want therefore to make a broader acknowledgement here of the incredible, essential, life-saving institution that is the NHS. The simple fact of the matter is that without it, my story – but so many others', too – would be very different, and much sadder.

Finally, most importantly, my family. As ever with the people who matter most, there aren't quite the right words, but I hope what I mean to say can be felt. My grandmother, Nancy, about whom I have written here, is an amazing woman, and I'm very grateful to have grown up next door to her, and for our ongoing correspondence later in life. To my mom and dad, Cynthia and Monte, I owe quite simply everything. Nothing I do would be possible without their unquestioning love, support, and friendship. I only hope I may someday be half as good a parent.

And to Xander: there's not a word in this book that I could have written without you. You make me a better writer, partner, daughter, friend, person. It feels too small a phrase, of course, but here it is, with all my love: thank you.

Sources of Quotations

On the Cusp

'conduit, a boundary, an exacting / course of thought' and 'Surface engraved with a narrow stroke', Matt Donovan, 'Line' (*Poetry*, 181, 5, March 2003, 333), available at: www.poetry foundation.org/poetrymagazine/browse?contentId=41776

'I had become interested in the more general problem of painting the water', David Hockney, *David Hockney by David Hockney*, ed. Nikos Stangos (London: Thames and Hudson, 1976), 100

'The Pacific still trembles in its bowl', Joan Didion, *South and West* (London: 4th Estate, 2017), 117

'as we flew in over Los Angeles, I looked down to see blue swimming pools', Christopher Simon Sykes, *Hockney: The Biography, Volume 1: 1937–1975* (London: Century, 2011), 142

'exists at different scales', Yi-Fu Tuan, *Space and Place* (Minneapolis: University of Minnesota Press, 1977), 149

'life-giving and murderous', Ivan Illich, H_2O *and the Waters of Forgetfulness* (London: Marion Boyars, 1986), 27 'a container, a box of right angles', Henning Eichberg, 'Body Culture as Paradigm', in John Bale and Chris Philo (eds.), *Body Cultures: Essays on Sport, Space and Identity* (London: Routledge, 1998), 151

'not as an external environment but as our own body', Yi-Fu Tuan, *Escapism* (Baltimore: Johns Hopkins University Press, 1998), 81

'you feel your body for what it mostly is', Roger Deakin, *Waterlog* (London: Vintage, 2000), 3

'shifting mirror', Ivan Illich, H_2o *and the Waters of Forgetfulness*, 25

'fantasies concerning the intra-uterine life', Sigmund Freud, *The Interpretation of Dreams* (Ware: Wordsworth Editions, 1997), 262

'the entire intrauterine existence of the higher mammals', Sándor Ferenczi, *Thalassa: A Theory of Genitality* (London: Karnac (Books) Ltd, 1989), 45

'the security and irresponsibility of the womb', Charles Sprawson, *Haunts of the Black Masseur: The Swimmer as Hero* (London: Vintage, 2013), 143

'Leaving behind the land, you go through the looking-glass surface', Roger Deakin, *Waterlog*, 3

'can cause a sense of detachment from ordinary life', Charles Sprawson, *Haunts of the Black Masseur*, 135

'But what if the "place" one wishes to escape from', Yi-Fu Tuan, *Escapism*, 31

'While the pool allows, even invites, intellectual wanderings', Thomas A.P. van Leeuwen, *The Springboard in the Pond: An Intimate History of the Swimming Pool* (Cambridge, MA, MIT Press, 1999), 7

'If there were even the slightest chance, Ester would think of nothing else', Lena Andersson, *Wilful Disregard* (London: Picador, 2016), 125

'A decision in the mind,' Sheila Heti, *Motherhood* (London: Harvill Secker, 2018), 30

A Wild Place

'I thought "I just want some other part of my body to hurt"', Donald McRae, 'Hannah Miley: Just Imagine What the Noise at the Olympics Will Be Like' (*Guardian*, 16 April 2012, available at: www.theguardian.com/sport/2012/apr/16/hannah-miley-olympics-london-2012-swimming)

'After twenty years I still search for the dumb focus I had as a competitive swimmer', Leanne Shapton, *Swimming Studies* (London: Penguin, 2012), 226

'a society built on quicksand', Pico Iyer, *The Global Soul* (London: Bloomsbury, 2001), 5

'one gets a sense of the body as a collection of numbers', Mark Greif, 'Against Exercise' (*n+1*, Issue 1, 2004, available at: www.nplusonemag.com/issue-1/essays/against-exercise/)

'the firm, developed body has become a symbol of correct attitude', Susan Bordo, *Unbearable Weight: Feminism, Western*

Culture, and the Body (Berkeley: University of California Press, 2003), 195

'is the means through which we experience and feel the world' and 'bodies are not only written upon', Tim Edensor, 'Walking in the British Countryside: Reflexivity, Embodied Practices and Ways to Escape' (*Body & Society* 6: 3–4, pp. 81–106, 2000; 100)

'The poles of the earth have wandered', John McPhee, *Basin and Range* (New York: Farrar, Straus and Giroux, 1981), 3

'about the rate at which our fingernails grow' and 'the present is not some kind of achieved terminus', Doreen Massey, *For Space* (London: Sage, 2005), 137

'the geography closest in', Adrienne Rich, 'Notes Toward a Politics of Location', in *Blood, Bread and Poetry: Selected Prose 1979–1985* (New York: W. W. Norton, 1986), 212

'the body is re-created so that it works better', John Bale, *Sports Geography* (London: Routledge, 2003), 8

'the honour of physical decline' and 'I don't care about the time I run', Haruki Murakami, *What I Talk About When I Talk About Running* (London: Vintage, 2009), 121

'To give birth is to be in a wild place' and 'And in the end, we won't have to go out and find the wild', Kathleen Jamie, 'A Lone Enraptured Male' (*London Review of Books* 30: 5 (6 March), 2008, available at: www.lrb.co.uk/v30/no5/kathleen-jamie/a-lone-enraptured-male)

'I think about loving swimming the way you love a country', Leanne Shapton, *Swimming Studies*, 320

Under the Surface

'Your body must be heard', Hélène Cixous, 'The Laugh of the Medusa' (*Signs* 1: 4, pp. 875–893, Summer 1976; 880

'happiness floats', Naomi Shihab Nye, 'So Much Happiness', *The Words Under the Words: Selected Poems* (Portland, Oregon: Eighth Mountain Press, 1998), 88

'Language is always late for its subject', Robert Macfarlane, *Landmarks* (London: Hamish Hamilton, 2015), 10

'in our hands', Maurice Merleau-Ponty, *Phenomenology of Perception* (London: Routledge, 2012), 145

'how to represent perception in language', Robert Macfarlane, *Landmarks*, 75

'I take the water in my arms' and 'my body becomes the ready instrument', Paul Valéry, *Cahiers/Notebooks, Volume 2* (Oxford: Peter Lang, 2000), 372–373

'Water is speaking', Nan Shepherd, *The Living Mountain* (London: Canongate, 2011), 22

'I try to work out how the water wants to hold me' and 'I don't need someone to tell me that my stroke looks great', Ian Thorpe and Robert Wainwright, *This Is Me: The Autobiography* (London: Simon & Schuster, 2012), xi–xii

'under me the central core of fire' and 'Slowly I have found my way in' and 'If I had other senses', Nan Shepherd, *The Living Mountain*, 105

'The most vital thing that can be listened to here', Nan Shepherd, *The Living Mountain*, 96

'call to mind an entire complex of sensations' and 'the cortex with its vast memory store', Yi-Fu Tuan, *Topophilia* (New Jersey: Prentice-Hall, 1974), 10

'The great object of life is Sensation', Lord Byron, in Leslie Marchand (ed.), *Lord Byron: Selected Letters and Journals* (Cambridge, MA: Belknap Press of Harvard University Press, 1982), 66

'fatal element', Thomas Medwin, *The Life of Percy Bysshe Shelley, Volume 1* (London: Thomas Cautley Newby, 1847), 177

'far advanced in pregnancy', *The Times* (12 December 1816), 2

'like some watcher of the skies', John Keats, 'On First Looking into Chapman's Homer', in Helen Gardner (ed.), *The New Oxford Book of English Verse* (Oxford: Clarendon Press, 1972), 563

'silent with swimming sense', Samuel Taylor Coleridge, 'This Lime-Tree Bower My Prison', in Morchard Bishop (ed.), *The Complete Poems of Samuel Taylor Coleridge* (London: Macdonald & Co., 1954), 159

'in terms of history silence was forgetting', Rachel Cusk, *Outline* (London: Faber & Faber, 2018), 245

'Perhaps silence can actually be read as a form of writing', Kate Zambreno, *Appendix Project* (Pasadena: Semiotext(e), 2019), 13

The Canyon

'I worry that I am disappearing', Emilie Pine, *Notes to Self* (London: Penguin, 2019), 39

'the pregnant body in public', Maggie Nelson, *The Argonauts* (London: Melville House, 2015), 112

'save her beauty from the Air', Charles Cotton, 'Winter', *Poems on Several Occasions* (London, 1689), 62

'These masks offered new possibilities', Christoph Heyl, 'When they are veyl'd on purpose to be seene: the Metamorphosis of the Mask in Seventeenth-and-Eighteenth-Century London', in Joanne Entwistle and Elizabeth Wilson (eds.), *Body Dressing* (Oxford: Berg, 2001), 127

'Not to fasten your Eyes upon any Person', Anonymous, 'Rules of Behaviour', *London Magazine* (February 1734), 66 (cited in Christoph Heyl, 'When they are veyl'd . . .', 128)

'If you made it understood that you were incognito', Christoph Heyl, 'When they are veyl'd . . .', 128

'constrains the way the physical body is perceived', Mary Douglas, *Natural Symbols* (London: Routledge, 2003), 65

'perhaps means that the body that is shown or hidden in smart clothes', John Harvey, 'Showing and Hiding: Equivocation in the Relations of Body and Dress' (*Fashion Theory* 11: 1, pp. 65–94, 2007; 81)

'we are all onions', Daniel Miller, *Stuff* (Cambridge: Polity Press, 2010), 13

'Another person's pregnancy', Nell Frizzell, *The Panic Years* (London: Bantam Press, 2021), 53

'Don't weep for me' and 'survived by ten nephews and nieces', Richard Severo, 'Gertrude Ederle, the First Woman to Swim Across the English Channel, Dies at 98' (*The New York Times*, 1 Dec 2003, available at: www.nytimes.com/2003/12/01/sports/gertrude-ederle-the-first-woman-to-swim-across-the-english-channel-dies-at-98.html)

'When in 1926 Gertrude Ederle became the first woman to swim the Channel', Charles Sprawson, *Haunts of the Black Masseur: The Swimmer as Hero* (London: Vintage, 2013), 262

'MOTHER OF 2 WILL MAKE ANOTHER TRY' and 'I think no woman is at her best', *Clearfield Progress*, 24 August 1926, cited in Gavin Mortimer, *The Great Swim* (London: Short Books, 2009), 30

'hard season', Maggie Nelson, *The Argonauts* (London: Melville House, 2015), 42

'a particularly dysfunctional moment', Ibid, 43

'It was an extraordinary moment' and 'I was grateful to him, relieved, giddy with pleasure', Leonard Michaels, *Sylvia* (New York: Farrar, Straus and Giroux, 2007), 48

An Inscription

'How we spend our days', Annie Dillard, *The Writing Life* (HarperCollins, 1990), 32

'Pregnancy begins as speculation', Joanne O'Leary, 'Portraying Pregnancy' (*London Review of Books* 42: 7, available at www.lrb.co.uk/the-paper/v42/n07/joanne-o-leary/at-the-foundling-museum)

'preserves its meaning by sinking deeply', Sally Ann Ness, 'The Inscription of Gesture; Inward Migrations in Dance', in Sally Ann Ness and Carrie Noland (eds.), *Migrations of Gesture* (Minneapolis: University of Minnesota, 2008), 4

'once the body's connective tissues', Sally Ann Ness, 'The Inscription of Gesture', 12

'it is a place-seeking, not a place-being, "in"' and 'Inscriptive gestures can be thought of as gestures that write something', Sally Ann Ness, 'The Inscription of Gesture', 1

'And what a dynamic, handsome object', Gaston Bachelard, *The Poetics of Space* (Boston: Beacon Press, 1994), 11

'the habits of a landscape', Robert Macfarlane, *The Old Ways* (London: Penguin, 2013), 17

'Through living in it, the landscape becomes a part of us', Tim Ingold, *The Perception of the Environment: Essays in Livelihood, Dwelling and Skill* (London: Routledge, 2000), 191

'Landscape can change the body encountering it', J.D. Dewsbury, 'Non-representational Landscapes and the Performative Affective Forces of Habit: From "Live" to "Blank"' (*Cultural Geographies* 22: 1, pp. 29–47, 2015; 36)

A Bright Spot

'reflects only part of the information back', Katie Paterson, 'Earth-Moon-Earth (Moonlight Sonata Reflected from the Surface of the Moon)' (available at: www.katiepaterson.org/portfolio/earth-moon-earth/)

'I think it's really important that there is still a place for the unknown' and 'The unknown point', Katie Paterson, exhibition: A place that exists only in moonlight: Katie Paterson & JMW Turner (26 Jan–6 May 2019, Turner Contemporary, Margate, UK)

'Did you see my little stillborn children', Robert Macfarlane, *Underland* (London: Hamish Hamilton, 2019), 16

'deep subterranean fact', Elaine Scarry, *The Body in Pain* (Oxford: Oxford University Press, 1985), 3

'everything is burning', Matt Lee (@APDiploWriter), '"Everything is burning, nothing will remain from the frame," Notre-Dame spokesman André Finot. "The Latest: #NotreDame spire collapses, interior in flames"' [Twitter post], 7.18 p.m., 15 April 2019 (available at: www.twitter.com/apdiplowriter/status/1117854617235116032?lang=en)

'I wanted to follow the rain on its meanderings', Roger Deakin, *Waterlog* (London: Vintage, 2000), 1

'I fear that without children it doesn't look like you have made a choice', Sheila Heti, *Motherhood* (London: Harvill Secker, 2018), 160–161

'like a diagnosis, a story can become a prison', Sarah Moss, *The Tidal Zone* (London: Granta, 2016), 329

'*Chiel, adrift*', Julia Copus, 'Pledge', *The World's Two Smallest Humans*, (London: Faber & Faber, 2012), 52

'listen I love you joy is coming', Kim Addonizio, 'To the Woman Crying Uncontrollably in the Next Stall' (*Diode* 9: 1, Spring 2016, available at: www.diodepoetry.com/v9n1/content/addonizio_k.html)

Endnotes

1　See for example 'How common is miscarriage?', Tommy's, www.tommys.org/pregnancy-information/im-pregnant/early-pregnancy/how-common-miscarriage.

2　'Women are 50% more likely than men to be given incorrect diagnosis following a heart attack', The BHF, 30 August 2016, www.bhf.org.uk/what-we-do/news-from-the-bhf/news-archive/2016/august/women-are-50-per-cent-more-likely-than-men-to-be-given-incorrect-diagnosis-following-a-heart-attack; Eliane Glaser, 'Invisible Women by Caroline Criado Perez – a world designed for men', *Guardian*, 28 February 2019, www.theguardian.com/books/2019/feb/28/invisible-women-by-caroline-criado-perez-review; Caroline Criado Perez, *Invisible Women* (London: Chatto & Windus, 2019).

3　'Overview: Ectopic pregnancy', NHS, www.nhs.uk/conditions/ectopic-pregnancy/.

4　'In vitro fertilisation (IVF)', Human Fertilisation & Embryology Authority, www.hfea.gov.uk/treatments/explore-all-treatments/in-vitro-fertilisation-ivf/.

5　'Acupuncture and success of IVF', NHS, 8 February 2008, www.nhs.uk/news/pregnancy-and-child/acupuncture-and-success-of-ivf/.